PRAISE FOR *EXHALE* AND RICHIE BOSTOCK

"This book will show you that there is a lot more to breathing than you think! Read it and learn Breathwork to strengthen and improve your physical, mental, and emotional well-being. Richie has gathered a wealth of knowledge and skills from some of the best Breathwork teachers in the world. And he has put together his own simple yet powerful set of exercises and techniques that will quickly have you breathing better, feeling better, and performing better! Take his breathing tests. Learn what kind of breather you are. Practice the exercises to increase mobility and flexibility in your spine and torso. Follow his brilliant twenty-minute 'daily routine' for twenty-one days and you will be amazed at the benefits! *Exhale* is an outstanding contribution to the art and science of Breathwork from a genuine student of the breath and an avid student of life. I highly recommend it!"

—Dan Brulé, author of the international bestseller
*Just Breathe: Mastering Breathwork for Success
in Life, Love, Business, and Beyond*

"Richie has a deep, experiential understanding of Breathwork. As with all the best teachers, his passion for conscious breathing techniques and his determination to bring them to a wider audience stem from his own personal journey. He conveys the practical ideas behind many different breathing disciplines in an easy, engaging way, allowing more people to access the potential of healthy breathing for life-changing health and resilience. Highly recommended!"

—Patrick McKeown, author of *The Oxygen Advantage*

"A fantastic guide to one of the most important exercises we've completely forgotten about. This book will help you refine the life enhancing practice of simply breathing properly."

—Dr. Rupy Aujla, MBBS, BSc, MRCGP,
founder of The Doctor's Kitchen

"A book that will literally transform lives mentally and physically for years to come by simply learning the impact of the breath—for me personally, having a lung disease (cystic fibrosis!) and being an athlete, this is an essential tool kit to not only improve my health and impact my life positivity, but also my performance in ultra endurance. An educational but inspiring book that had me hooked from the first line, one I'll be reading time and time again, which includes everyday practices to improve the way I breathe, enable me to control stress, and improve my sleep. Richie really is building a legacy one breath at a time—it's truly powerful and empowering."
—Sophie Grace Holmes, coach and ultra-endurance athlete

"Richie is an extraordinary individual, dedicated to facilitating deep healing and transformation. He has a strong intuition and is committed to the guidance of human flourishing through development of community and collaboration with trusted expertise. My personal experience of Breathwork with Richie has been life changing. I truly began to see that within us all there is the possibility for deep peace and connection."
—Dr. Tamsin Lewis, founder of Wellgevity,
holistic and personalized medical
service to guide your health span

"I've participated in breath work with Richie in groups, one-on-one, and in online sessions and am delighted that he is now offering the benefits of his knowledge, wisdom, and kindness to the world in the form of this book. *Exhale* is your comprehensive guide to understanding what type of breather you are, guiding you toward a more fulfilling life by simply changing the way you breathe. Amazing!"
—Dr. Zoe Williams, MBBS, DRCOG, MRCGP

PENGUIN BOOKS

EXHALE

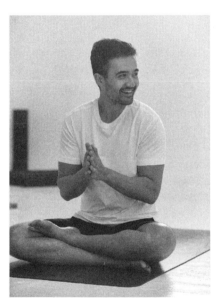

Richie Bostock is one of the world's leading practitioners in Breathwork, having spent years traveling across five continents learning from many of the modern-day masters in the discipline. Currently, he holds workshops and retreats across the world and works with large organizations such as Google, Unilever, and Ernst & Young. He continues to work one-on-one with athletes, fitness influencers, and high-profile clients and regularly partners with leading fitness brands such as Lululemon.

Exhale

40 BREATHWORK EXERCISES
TO HELP YOU FIND YOUR CALM,
SUPERCHARGE YOUR HEALTH,
AND PERFORM AT YOUR BEST

Richie Bostock

life

PENGUIN BOOKS
An imprint of Penguin Random House LLC
penguinrandomhouse.com

First published in Great Britain by Penguin Life, a part of
Penguin Random House UK, 2020
Published in Penguin Books 2020

LIBRARY OF CONGRESS CATALOGING-IN-PUBLICATION CONTROL NUMBER: 2020943824 (PRINT)

ISBN 9780143135326 (paperback)
ISBN 9780525506997 (ebook)

Printed in the United States of America
10 9 8 7 6 5 4 3 2 1

Set in Avenir LT Pro

Contents

For my parents, Yujin and David;

this book exists because of you

"Then the Lord God formed man from the dust of the ground and breathed the breath of life into his nostrils, and the man became a living being . . ."

Genesis 2:7

". . . and then man forgot."

Richie Bostock

EXHALE

Introduction:
Change your breath, change your life

Have you ever asked yourself why you breathe? You may think this question has a pretty obvious answer—we need to breathe to survive! But is there more to breathing than simply to bring oxygen into your body?

You breathe somewhere between 17,000 and 29,000 times per day, or 6 to 10 million breaths per year. If you did anything else that often, you'd probably have a pretty good idea how and why you did it. So it always surprises me how little understanding there is about this essential act of living that we do every moment of every day.

In fact, most of us are so unaware of our breathing that we don't notice how, either over time or even in a single moment, we can develop dysfunctional breathing habits that are slowly destroying our health and happiness, manifesting in physical and mental symptoms from fatigue, headaches, digestive issues, and sleep disorders to chronic stress and anxiety.

It is estimated that roughly 60 percent of all emergency ambulance calls in larger American cities involve breath-related disorders.[1] To quote Donna Farhi, a world-renowned yoga instructor, "A casual glance of any city street will reveal the extent to which tight belts, tight bodies, and tight schedules are literally taking our breath away."

But there is good news. Watch how a toddler breathes, and notice the open and flowing nature of their breath. With some understanding and practice, you can easily retrain your own breathing mechanics back to their original and optimal state. It's just like learning any new skill. And this book is here to help you do just that.

And it doesn't stop there. Think of the breath as your body's very own built-in Swiss Army knife. Here, you have a tool that can help you in so many situations, and improve your physical and mental health and performance and emotional well-being. You might be a sleep-deprived parent, a stressed business executive, an elite athlete, or anyone in between. By simply learning how to use your breath as a tool, the way nature intended you to, you will experience dramatic changes in your life. Think about it—if this promise is as simple as taking a few breaths in a certain way, what are you waiting for?

So, what I present to you in this book is the essential knowledge and techniques from my years of learning and working with the breath. I've distilled the expertise from many modern Breathwork masters, elite athletic trainers, psychologists, therapists, researchers, doctors, and health practitioners into a simple, step-by-step guide for you to start to breathe with purpose.

I believe this knowledge, stemming from both ancient wisdom and scientific innovation, should be known by everyone. We all breathe, after all. This book serves as a starting point to help you unleash the full power and potential of your breath. You already have it, so you might as well start using it!

I start out in **Chapter 1** with the sole intention of inspiring you to consider this the start of your own exploration into a whole new world of exciting possibility.

As a young child, I loved any book, movie, or TV show about a person who had extraordinary abilities. From movies about superheroes gifted with supernatural strength or speed, to books about wizards and witches who could perform incredible magic, I loved the idea that people have secret powers beyond belief. I think secretly I was hoping that one day I would tap into some dormant superpower that was just waiting to be revealed.

Years later and I still can't fly or lift mountains. However, in **Chapter 1** you'll discover how an interesting turn of events in my life took me on a path of exploration to discover and research a real-life superpower that, as it turns out, is something that everyone has in their possession, but very few people actually know how to use. A superpower that can:

- Give you more natural energy than your next espresso.
- Help you to think more clearly and be more creative.
- Turn off your busy mind and find calm, even in the most stressful situations.

- Access meditative flow states in a matter of minutes (even if you have never meditated before).
- Increase your athletic endurance.
- Help you to sleep better.
- And make you feel blissfully happy.

Sounds pretty incredible, right? Well, you already have it, waiting to be unleashed, and it's quite literally right under your nose.

In **Chapter 2**, I'll teach you about different breathing habits and behaviors and give you the steps you can take to assess your own breathing, to see if you are doing it correctly!

In **Chapter 3**, based on your assessment, you'll be provided with a bespoke 21-day *Breathe Right* program that will completely transform and optimize your breathing habits.

The rest of the book is dedicated to providing you with the best Breathwork techniques and strategies that I've experienced and developed that you can easily implement into your own life.

Chapter 4 offers you the essential techniques for everyday use. But it doesn't stop there. In **Chapter 5**, you'll find a vast range of techniques to help you in a variety of situations: from easing panic attacks, increasing athletic performance and relieving hangovers, to increasing sexual pleasure and aiding in the treatment of many chronic ailments and diseases. Ultimately, you'll have a variety of techniques ready to use for whatever suits your life and your unique situation.

You begin life with your first breath. You leave life with your last. How you breathe in between can profoundly impact your experience. This book will explain why, and show you how to breathe with purpose.

Old and new worlds collide: Ancient wisdom meets modern science

Breathing is the only function in our body that happens completely automatically and is 100 percent under our control. This is not an accident of nature, it's a human design feature.

Many ancient traditions knew this, and developed practices based around breathing to increase the quality of their physical, mental, and emotional health.

The well-known yogic discipline of pranayama is a system of breathing exercises designed to work with what the Hindu sages referred to as Prana, or life-force energy.

Many other cultures around the world—such as the Tibetans, Sufis, Taoists and shamanic societies—developed their own sacred breathing techniques, as a way to improve their state of being or even to enter visionary states for spiritual experiences.

The importance of the breath as an essential element in one's state of being was even highlighted in some of the oldest languages. In ancient Greek, the word for soul, "psyche pneuma," also means breath. In Latin, "anima spiritus" also means soul and breath.

In modern times, the breath has been forgotten, taken for granted and swept aside as something that "just happens" to keep us alive.

But now, as science continues to advance, more and more research supports what ancient traditions have known for centuries: that the way we breathe significantly impacts our quality of life.

Mental health professionals have pioneered the use of breathing techniques as an effective form of emotional therapy, helping people work through mental and emotional challenges such as trauma, anxiety, and depression.

More and more athletes and sports teams are adopting breathing practices to gain an edge. To improve output, elite endurance athletes match the cadence of their step, stroke, or pedal to their breathing. Professional boxers and mixed martial arts fighters use breathing techniques in between rounds, to recover as quickly as possible, get ready for the next round. All these techniques, ancient and modern, are Breathwork.

To quote Dr. Andrew Weil, celebrity doctor and world leader in integrative medicine:

"If I had to limit my advice on healthier living to just one tip, it would be to simply learn how to breathe correctly."

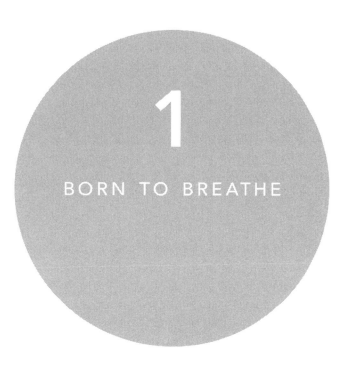

1

BORN TO BREATHE

As I step off the ice and enter the zero-degree water, a thousand hypodermic needles seem to simultaneously pierce my skin. Electricity jolts through my nervous system, slamming me into "fight, flight, or freeze" mode. Every muscle in my body has no choice but to tense up. I can barely breathe. But I'm not the only one.

The Wim Hof Method (WHM) instructor tells me to do my best to relax, to focus on my breath and breathe deeply and slowly. Once I'm able to catch my breath again and slow it down, the cold no longer feels quite so bad. I relax, letting go of each tense muscle, one by one, until I feel like a jellyfish floating among the ice. Each time I re-enter the water, I just focus on my breathing, relaxing and surrendering into the moment. Although the cold is never pleasant, it becomes strangely bearable.

Let me tell you how I got here.

For as long as I can remember, I've always had a fascination with trying to find answers to the big questions of life. What is the nature of reality? How did the universe come to be and why do we exist in it? I would often ask my parents these questions, hoping for answers. However, the most consistent response I received back was, "You think too much." By the time I was eighteen, I had already read, watched, and listened to hours and hours of material on philosophy, spirituality, psychology, and personal growth. Yet when I reached my midtwenties, I still felt like I was no closer to getting answers to any of my questions, which left me unsatisfied and unhappy.

I'd been working at an international consulting firm in Australia for nearly six years, with big visions of career progression, traveling the world, and enjoying all the material successes of working in a big firm. While I enjoyed some of the work and got along well with my colleagues, it became clear over the years of caffeine-fueled late nights in the office that doing eighty-hour workweeks under fluorescent lights was not what I was supposed to be doing on this planet.

One of the greatest blessings I've received in my life is my parents, who are always ready to listen and give support where they can. After confiding my struggles to them, they gave me some sage advice: to take some time off work, leave my current routine and environment, and go somewhere completely different to clear my head. When you feel lost or stuck in a rut, getting distance from your regular environment allows you to leave the old patterns of thinking and feeling behind, making it easier to more clearly identify the problem points and what needs to change. This advice proved to be the turning point for the rest of my life to begin.

It just so happened that a good friend of mine had recently returned from a trip volunteering at orphanages in Peru. One evening we had dinner together and he shared many stories about his experiences. As he spoke, something inside me was telling me that this kind of experience of service to others in a different part of the world, in a different culture, was exactly the thing I should do at this stage of my life. I asked if he would help me arrange to volunteer at the same orphanages that he had worked at. Luckily, my boss agreed for me to take an indefinite sabbatical from my work and, in nine days, I was on a plane to Peru.

While on the plane, the anxiety of stepping into the complete unknown, leaving everything that I knew and was familiar with behind, hit me like a sledgehammer. My heart felt like it was about to beat out of my chest and I noticed how my breathing became rapid and erratic as my mind raced with all sorts of doubts, worries, and questions about what the hell I was doing. Despite this, my gut was telling me that this moment in my life would be like a crossroads and that, when I got back, nothing would be the same. This was a terrifying feeling, but I decided to surrender to it and embrace it. As I was going to a place where nobody knew me, this was an opportunity to put aside everything that I thought I knew about myself and start afresh.

I ended up spending nearly three months in Peru, volunteering and traveling around the country. The experience was transformative. Given the opportunity to be completely myself, without the expectations of people in my usual environment, I unfolded into a completely different person. Each morning, I'd wake up and say to myself, "Forget who you think you are!" By letting go of any ideas on how I would or should normally be, I'd often surprise myself at how differently I started to think, feel, or act. Even the way I laughed changed!

Yet I knew that when I returned to my normal environment, I'd be under pressure to slip back into the old ways that had led to my unhappiness. (How many times have you gone on vacation and received inspiration to do something when you got home, but once you got back you forgot all about it?) Now, having reconnected with a part of myself that had long been ignored, my intuition was telling me that I was going to have to make some very big changes. And that if I didn't do it quickly, I might succumb to my old ways.

In a moment of inspiration (or was it desperation?), within ten days of arriving home I quit my job, ended a long-term relationship, sold everything I owned except for a suitcase of clothes, and decided I wanted to leave Australia and move overseas. My parents were living in Hong Kong at the time and suggested I could stay with them until I worked out what my next move would be. With no better ideas, I moved to Hong Kong.

I really had no plan, no idea what I was doing. But I trusted my intuition and surrendered to the unknown. Again following my gut, I decided that I wanted to learn how to build websites and mobile apps. This ended up being an inspired decision.

Working for myself as a web developer gave me the flexibility for the journey that was about to come.

It was during this time that my family received some news that would rock us to the core. My dad was diagnosed with multiple sclerosis (MS), an autoimmune disease that slowly breaks down the body's nervous system, with no cure. What was particularly scary for us was that my grandmother also had MS, so our family had already seen firsthand how the disease can cripple someone. However, until the day she left us, my grandmother was the strongest and most positive person that I have ever met, and I still think of her whenever I need strength.

Since there was no set treatment plan for MS, my mom and I would scour the internet for any information or advice on anything that could be useful for Dad, from alternative treatments to lifestyle changes. It always amazes me how just one book, documentary, or podcast can completely change the course of your life. This is exactly what happened to me.

One day I was listening to a podcast, an interview with a man named Wim Hof, a fascinating Dutch man commonly referred to as "the Iceman." He holds more than twenty world records related to cold exposure activities, including staying submerged in an ice bath for close to two hours and climbing Mount Everest to an altitude of about 22,000 feet, wearing only shorts.

In this podcast, Wim talked about a method he'd developed through his own experiences that was fantastic for anyone's physical and mental health. But what caught my attention was his specific point that the method was effective in helping people with autoimmune diseases, including MS. Intrigued, I started to research exactly what the Wim Hof Method (WHM) was all about. I discovered that it was based on two main elements: cold exposure activities, such as cold showers and ice baths; and breathing techniques. Could something as simple as taking a cold shower and doing specific breathing techniques every day really help my dad? I was excited.

With nothing to lose, I spoke to my dad the next day to see if he wanted to try it. The conversation went something like this:

Me: Hey, Dad.

Dad: Hey, Rich.

Me: Check this out. This Dutch guy called "the Iceman" says that if you take a cold shower and breathe every day, it will really help you with your MS.

[Silence.]

Dad: Are you suggesting that taking cold showers and breathing a bit will cure my MS?

Me: Well . . . yeah . . .

[Longer silence.]

Me: Oh, um, never mind.

Looking back, I can see how I was coming across as absolutely insane, suggesting that breathing and a bit of cold water could tackle a problem that modern medical practices hadn't been able to fix! But for some reason my intuition was screaming at me, saying this was important. After a little more research, I discovered I could attend a week-long WHM training course in Poland during the winter. I would learn the technique and do all the crazy cold-related stunts that Wim did. So I decided to send myself on a reconnaissance mission. I'd go to Poland and find out what this was really about. If I found it useful, maybe Dad would be more willing to try it for himself one day.

> *Three months later, I find myself standing barefoot on the ice, at the foot of a frozen-over waterfall in Poland. It's 21 degrees Fahrenheit. I'm wearing only shorts and trying really hard to not die. The WHM instructor facilitating this part of the training tells us that we're going to do an exercise where we submerge ourselves in the thirty-two-degree water for a few minutes, then come out and try to warm up naturally, using a series of movements he calls "horse stance," while still standing, soaking wet, on the ice. And we aren't just going to do this once, or twice, but three times in a row.*

> *After the third round of swimming in the ice water, I step back on to the ice and notice something very strange. I'm not cold. In fact, I feel boiling hot, like*

I'm back on a beach in Australia in the middle of summer. I've heard stories of lost mountain climbers later being found with all their clothes off. The first stage of hypothermia can be that you feel extremely hot, even though you're freezing to death. So, right away, my mind jumped to the worst conclusion. "Well, I guess that's it, I've got hypothermia. I'm going to be that guy that ruins the training for everyone!"

So I approach the closest WHM instructor and ask him, "I'm not cold, I think I'm starting to sweat— what's happening to me?" *The instructor gives me a big smile and says,* "Rich, look at your shoulders!" When I turn to look at my shoulders, *steam is coming off my back. I look back at my instructor, shocked. He simply proceeds to explain how the body is capable of so much more if we just let it. By focusing on relaxing and letting go in the ice water, the body is allowed to do whatever it needs to do to survive. Take Wim, himself. To keep his core body temperature stable during his stunts, he has been measured as increasing his metabolism by nearly 300 percent. Something similar has likely just happened to me.*

This was just one of the many perspective-shifting experiences I had during my week in Poland. We hiked wearing only shorts, barefoot in the snow that sometimes came up to our knees. We even climbed the tallest mountain in Poland, braving whipping wind and snow, wearing only our shorts. At the top, it got down to -2 degrees.

These experiences in extreme cold were incredible, but for me the most profound moment of the entire training was on the first day, when I experienced Breathwork for the very first time.

> *Breathwork is when you intentionally become aware of your breath and use it to improve your physical and mental health and performance and emotional well-being.*

I'll come back to this definition later. For now, let me tell you that you will never forget the first time you do a deep Breathwork session. I didn't.

As a group, we went down into the basement of the hotel where we were staying. We lay down on the ground and, for about forty-five minutes, performed a sequence of breathing techniques aimed at creating big changes to our physiology and big shifts in how we thought and felt.

Whether it was the physical sensations of buzzing and vibration through the body or the experience of various emotional states—from bliss and euphoria to feelings of power and strength—for me, it was like nothing I had ever experienced in my life.

After the session was over, I was filled with such a sense of peace, clarity, and confidence that my life was exactly where it needed to be and that everything was going to be perfect. It was as though every doubting thought had been silenced, leaving only a blissful sense of calm. I remember asking myself, *"How is it possible that I can feel this good just by breathing? Why doesn't everybody know about this?"* Little did I know that the first seed had been planted of what would direct my life for many years to come.

After returning from Poland, I showed Dad the photos and shared stories of my experience. He agreed to try it. Today, my dad practices Breathwork and takes cold showers daily. This, in combination with a change in diet, has stopped any progression in his MS for years.

My experience in Poland, and seeing how breathing was helping my dad, ignited a passion in me to find out what else people were doing using their breath. Over the following years, I traveled the world to seek the teachings of anyone who was doing something interesting with breathing. My fascination has taken me across five continents, spending time and learning with yogis, Breathwork masters, doctors, researchers, therapists, physical therapists, and elite athletic coaches.

I've continued to witness the transformative effects of what happens when people learn to use their breathing as a tool to create massive change in their physical, mental, and emotional states. That's what we call Breathwork.

What is Breathwork?

When I teach classes and workshops, I always start by asking who has done Breathwork before. Usually, a smattering of hands will go up and I'll ask them what they have done. The responses often vary from:

- *"I do yoga and there's lots of breathing in that."*
- *"I'm a singer/actor and we focus a lot on how we breathe."*
- *"I do tai chi or qi gong."*
- *"I've done really, really long and intense breathing sessions for emotional healing."*
- *"When I go scuba diving, I really have to focus on my breathing."*
- *"I mean, I breathe every day, so does that count?"*

As you can see, people define Breathwork in lots of different ways and there are many schools/institutions that will claim other definitions of Breathwork. So let me return to the very simple and straightforward definition of what I believe Breathwork to be:

> *Breathwork is when you intentionally become aware of your breath and use it to improve your physical and mental health and performance and emotional well-being.*

This definition encapsulates all the different techniques and methods where your breath is the primary focus—from simple three-minute techniques that help you feel relaxed, to daily breathing practices that can help to relieve chronic back pain, to practices that can induce peak performance states and meditative flow states, to techniques to improve sports performance and methods for deep healing.

This means there are hundreds of applications of Breathwork and thousands of different techniques. Regardless of who you are and what you do, one or many forms of Breathwork is an essential tool for fulfilling your potential in becoming the happiest, healthiest, and highest-performing version of you!

Now I know this can seem pretty overwhelming. After all, the way we breathe is central to just about every part of life. To simplify things, let me share with you how I categorize all the different types of Breathwork:

Five kinds of Breathwork

1. EVERYDAY BREATHWORK

Quick techniques you can use throughout the day to quickly change your state

Examples:

- Decrease stress, anxiety, and nervousness (pages 110–14 and 132–36)
- Create more energy (pages 108–9)
- Help to sleep (pages 116–21)

2. CORRECTIVE BREATHWORK

Techniques to correct your breathing mechanics to improve your day-to-day breathing

Examples:

- Learn to breathe diaphragmatically (pages 82–85)
- Increase thoracic flexibility (pages 66–79 and 88–90)

3. PERFORMANCE BREATHWORK

Techniques to help you perform better in a physically demanding activity

Examples:

- Increase athletic performance (pages 153–59)
- Speed up recovery (page 160)
- Improve singing, dancing, acting

4. MIND–BODY BREATHWORK

Techniques and practices to further improve your physical, mental and emotional health, and vitality

Examples:

- Pranayama (pages 106–7), Buteyko (page 167), Wim Hof Method (pages 178–92)
- Techniques for medical issues (pages 167–92)

5. INTEGRATIVE BREATHWORK

Methods of Breathwork for therapeutic purposes, healing and spiritual experience, and exploration

Examples:

- Rebirthing, Holotropic Breathwork, Transformational breathing, Biodynamic Breathwork (pages 195–201)

The journey of the breath

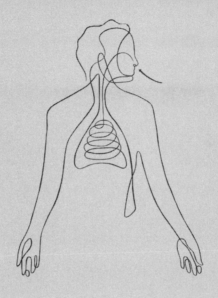

At the nose:

On a normal healthy inhale, you breathe in about 5–6 liters of air, usually consisting of 20.95 percent oxygen. This air is pulled through your nose or mouth into your windpipe, or trachea, which then splits into two branches called bronchi and further into bronchioles. The bronchioles then enter tiny air sacs in your lungs called alveoli.

At the lungs:

Depending on the size of your lungs, you can have anywhere between 300 million and 600 million alveoli, each of which is encased by tiny blood vessels called capillaries. If you stretched out the area of contact of your capillaries and alveoli, the surface area would easily be enough to cover an entire tennis court. It's here that the oxygen in the air you inhale passes into the bloodstream.

At the heart:

Oxygen-rich blood is transported through to the left side of your heart, then pumped through the aorta to all the other parts of your body via a complex labyrinth of vessels.

If all these arteries, veins, and capillary vessels of the human circulatory system were laid end to end, the total length would measure 60,000 miles. That's nearly two and a half times around the Earth.

In this way, oxygen is transported to each and every cell in your body for what is perhaps the single most important biochemical reaction that occurs inside you: cellular respiration.

At the cells:

Every one of the approximately 37 trillion cells that we are made up of is like a little power station. Cellular respiration is the process of how we create energy from what we eat and what we breathe in. This energy is what keeps our heart beating, our food digesting, creates electrical signals in our brain, and fuels our muscles to run, jump, or lift at our best.

At the nose:

Alongside energy, cellular respiration also creates carbon dioxide, which is transported through your bloodstream to the right side of your heart and pumped to your lungs to be expelled through your exhale.

2

WHAT KIND OF A
BREATHER ARE YOU?

The way you breathe is as unique as your fingerprint. You have your own personal breathing habits and behaviors that you've developed through the course of your life. If you are like most people, the events in your life and the effects of living in our modern society have unknowingly altered the open and flowing nature of your breath that you once had as a young child to a breathing pattern that is far more restricted. Why?

- *Tight trousers, belts, skirts, and dresses are literally suffocating us.*
- *An overly sedentary lifestyle of sitting in cars, buses, trains, and in front of computers results in muscle tightness through important postural and breathing muscles.*
- *Physical injuries can also create learned dysfunctional breathing habits, which can remain long after the injury has healed.*
- *Traumatic events and chronic stress can cause the body to get stuck in "fight, flight, or freeze" mode, forcing our breathing to adjust accordingly.*

- *Many of us unconsciously suck in our bellies, restricting the movement in our abdomen in an attempt to look slimmer and more attractive.*

In this chapter, you'll learn about the muscles we all use to breathe and the different ways that people actually use them. Toward the end of the chapter, you'll learn how to assess your own breathing to determine the kind of breather you are today.

Stop now, just for a second, and breathe naturally. What do you observe about your own breathing?

Breathing is movement. So you have to engage your muscles. Here's the thing—just as you're not consciously thinking about your hamstrings when you run, it's the same with the muscles you use to breathe. Unless, that is, you *choose* to focus your attention on how you breathe, in which case you can consciously control the engagement of these muscles.

Get acquainted with your primary breathing muscles

Breathing happens in your torso, that cylinder supported by your spine. Your 24 ribs, 12 on each side, connect to your spine and are flexible, enabling multiple directions of movement. How mobile and flexible you are in your torso has a big impact on how you breathe.

It's all about your diaphragm

When it comes to correct breathing, the only place to start is with your diaphragm. This most important muscle in the movement of breathing is fibrous and parachute-shaped. It separates your thoracic cavity—the space your heart and lungs occupy—from the abdominal cavity, where your digestive organs live. It attaches to your spine, the lower ribs, and the bottom of your sternum.

Now, the movement of your diaphragm is controlled by the phrenic nerve, which runs all the way from your neck to your diaphragm.

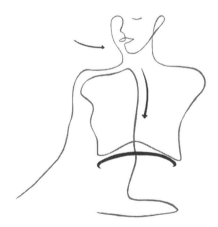

Inhaling . . . your diaphragm contracts and descends, pulling air into the lowest parts of your lungs.

Exhaling . . . your diaphragm relaxes and ascends, forcing the inhaled air out of your lungs.

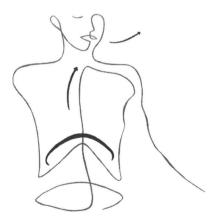

What you get is an up-and-down motion that massages and stimulates your internal organs. With your liver, stomach, and large intestine sitting directly below your diaphragm, this massage is excellent for digestion. Even your kidneys, at the back of your torso, benefit directly from the motion of your diaphragm. This pushing-down motion on your organs is why diaphragmatic breathing is often referred to as "belly breathing." As the diaphragm descends, your organs underneath are pushed to the front, back, and sides. This causes your abdomen to expand, giving the appearance of breathing into the stomach.

Not forgetting the muscles in your ribs and back

Between your ribs, you have intercostal muscles moving in concert with your diaphragm. When you inhale, they contract to pull your ribcage both upward and outward. When you exhale, they relax to reduce the space in your thoracic cavity. You also have some deep back muscles—the levatores costarum—running down along the thoracic area of your spine. These help to lift your ribcage when you breathe in.

Introducing your secondary breathing muscles

Your diaphragm, intercostals, and levatores are your primary breathing muscles. They're undoubtedly the endurance athletes of breathing, designed to run 24/7.

Now for your secondary breathing muscles—the sprinters, designed to work for short bursts of time when your body needs more oxygen and needs it now, like when you are exercising. They include muscles in your neck, upper chest, and back (omohyoid, sternocleidomastoid, scalenes, upper trapezius, rhomboids major and minor), as well as bigger muscles in your torso and abdomen (latissimus dorsi, quadratus lumborum, and superficial abdominal muscles).

These muscles are also engaged when you are stressed. Why? Because the changes that occur in our body when we feel stress are biologically preparing us to act in response to a physical threat, for example, to be able to run or fight off a bear. In these situations, the metabolic demands for oxygen are higher, therefore these secondary breathing muscles will kick in.

In modern times you don't usually have to worry about fighting off a bear; however, instead there are ever-present micro stressors, from worrying about work and career or financial stability to how many likes our photo received on Instagram. Regardless of the source of the stress, the body's stress response is the same, which means that many people are using their secondary breathing muscles all the time.

What is important to understand is that the relationship between your breath and your nervous system is a two-way street, so not only will your breathing respond to changes in how you are feeling, but the way you breathe can also affect how your nervous system fires in the first place. If you get into the habit of breathing using these muscles designed to be

INHALING

- Purpose: to bring air into lungs to ensure the consistent delivery of oxygen (O_2) to cells.
- In a relaxed state, initiated by diaphragm.
- Supported and aided by other primary breathing muscles expanding the thoracic cavity, allowing lungs to pull in air.
- When metabolic requirements rise during exercise, dormant secondary breathing muscles kick in to increase breathing speed and deliver more O_2.

used in times of fight or flight, your brain will interpret this as a sign of danger and increase the stress response. More stress, for no reason at all.

EXHALING

- Purpose: to expel air from lungs and to balance carbon dioxide (CO_2) levels.
- Primary breathing muscles relax.
- Thoracic cavity shrinks back to its neutral position, expelling air out of the lungs.
- When relaxed, the muscles are briefly at rest, providing a pause between the end of the exhale and the beginning of the next inhale.
- Speaking, singing, and shouting cause extra muscles to control the exhale, slowing it down or speeding it up.
- During exercise, exhaling becomes more forceful to rapidly expel CO_2 from the system.

Nose, or mouth?

One of the most common questions I receive is, *"Should I be breathing through my nose or my mouth?"* The answer is not simply one or the other, it actually depends. As a rule of thumb, get into the habit of breathing in and out through your nose—that's what it's for.

Think of your nose like an air-conditioner that filters, warms, and humidifies the air you inhale before it reaches your lungs. Nasal breathing increases oxygen delivery to your cells, keeps carbon dioxide levels in your blood balanced, and can even improve the overall capacity of your lungs. The nose creates more resistance to the inflowing air than breathing through your mouth, therefore slowing down your breathing rate and providing a more relaxing effect on your nervous system.[2]

Nasal breathing also helps to produce nitric oxide, an important gas whose antiviral and antibacterial qualities work on the destruction of viruses and parasites in the airways and lungs.

Nitric oxide also acts as a vasodilator, relaxing the muscles of blood vessels and causing them to widen, which helps with circulation. While important for everyone, an increase in circulation is particularly useful for athletes. Some even take sports supplements that help increase nitric oxide (see page 154).

It can, however, be useful to breathe through your mouth for short periods of time to create different effects in the body.

In this book, you'll find a number of different breathing techniques that demonstrate the effects of purposeful mouth breathing. But please note that these deliberate techniques are only for temporary use. Once you've done one, it's important to return to a regular breathing pattern of in and out through your nose.

Learn to spot different types of breather

Let me share with you a summary of the four most common types of breathing patterns I've observed: reverse breather; chest breather; belly breather; diaphragmatic breather. Which one do you most identify with? Perhaps you're a mix of several.

THE REVERSE BREATHER

When you inhale, you see . . .

- Your breath starts in the upper chest.
- Your shoulders rise.
- Your chest aggressively puffs out and upward.
- Your abdomen pulls in toward the spine.
- You may feel your muscles in your neck tense.

An optimal breath is one where you allow your diaphragm to fully descend on the inhale, pushing down on the organs beneath it and expanding your abdomen to the front, back, and sides.

On the exhale, your diaphragm relaxes and rises, enabling your organs to return back to their original position. As a result, your abdomen shrinks back to its resting formation.

When you are reverse breathing, however, this action sequence is reversed. On the inhale, you suck in your abdomen toward your spine. Then, on the exhale, your abdomen moves back outward. This means that, most of the time, your stomach muscles are contracted and both inhale and exhale are tightly controlled.

This habit of reversing the natural mechanics of breathing can exist for many reasons, from a past physical injury to emotional trauma.

THE CHEST BREATHER

When you inhale, you see . . .

- Your breath starts in the upper chest.
- Your shoulders rise.
- Your chest aggressively puffs out and upward.
- Your mid to lower ribs expand sideways.

- Your abdomen doesn't move, or only moves minimally following the chest.

If you're a chest breather, you're over-reliant on using secondary breathing muscles in your upper chest, back, and shoulders. This will often cause you stiffness, tension, and eventually pain in these areas.

As this type of breather, your stomach muscles are often chronically tense or braced, acting as a steel wall that won't allow your organs to move outward when you breathe in.

This is the most common breathing pattern I see. There are so many reasons why this habit can form: from sucking in your stomach to look slimmer, through to chronic stress.

THE BELLY BREATHER

When you inhale, you see . . .

- Movement starting in your belly.
- Your shoulders stay still.
- Your chest remains still.
- Your mid to lower ribs move minimally or not at all.
- Your stomach rises forcefully forward.
- The sides of your abdomen pull inward.

If you go to yoga classes, it's not uncommon for the teacher to tell you to "breathe into the belly" for a greater sense of calm. Although this is the first step to breathing correctly—especially if you're a reverse or chest breather—it isn't necessarily the correct way to breathe all the time.

As a result, you'll often focus really hard on breathing into your belly and start to engage the big secondary breathing muscles there (transverse abdominis, rectus abdominis, and internal and external obliques) to force your belly outward as you inhale. These muscles should not be initiating the breath but instead should stay relaxed and only move passively as a result of the movement of the primary breathing muscles.

This focused belly breathing will often cause the intercostal muscles between your ribs to disengage. As a result, your ribcage will become static, restricting the movement of your diaphragm.

THE DIAPHRAGMATIC BREATHER

When you inhale, you see . . .

- Movement beginning in your diaphragm around the bottom of your ribs.
- Your chest expanding, following the movement of your lower ribs.

- Your shoulders stay mostly still.
- Your mid to lower ribs expand sideways.
- Your abdomen rises passively, following the movement of your ribs.

This is the way nature intended us to breathe.

Watch any healthy child, dog, or cat breathe and you'll instantly recognize this breathing pattern.

People will often say that just watching someone breathe in this natural and relaxed style brings a sense of relaxation and can even be hypnotizing.

Have you identified a particular form of breathing pattern in yourself, yet? Well, let me tell you now that it's possible for you to exhibit other breathing behaviors that can coexist alongside these more common breathing patterns. Here are some of the more irregular behaviors of breathing that I frequently observe:

The no-breather

As a no-breather, you're not going to optimally inhale or exhale. Instead, your breath hovers in limbo between the two, as you take small sips of air, often at quite a fast rate, breathing into your chest.

This usually happens due to muscular tension throughout your thorax and abdomen, suppressing the rising motion of breathing in. There's very little movement throughout your body. Sometimes, as the name suggests, this form of breathing is barely noticeable.

I've often seen a high correlation between this breathing behavior and feelings of fear. Perhaps the fear of being noticed or seen, the fear of not being good enough, or not feeling safe as a result of trauma or abuse. It's often a physical manifestation of deeper issues.

The breath-holder

This is a familiar breathing type to many people. You're sitting at your desk, writing an e-mail to your boss, updating her on your work progress. Suddenly, you realize you're not breathing! So you take in a big gasp of air. You've just experienced "e-mail apnoea," a term credited to former Apple executive Linda Stone, describing unknowingly going without breathing for extended periods of time. If this is you, don't worry, you're not alone. Just ask your fellow employees if they've experienced this before. You may be surprised how prevalent it is.

Unconscious breath-holding appears to be a reflex in response to a stressor or threat. Whether real or imagined, you're anticipating an outcome or simply waiting for something to happen.

There are some instances where conscious breath-holding is perfectly acceptable and even useful. During movements of exertion (e.g., lifting weights), holding your breath during certain points of the movement can be encouraged. However, if you find yourself consistently unconsciously holding your breath when at rest, this would be something to pay attention to.

If you believe you're a breath-holder, start to become aware of the moments when it happens. Then ask yourself the following questions and look for insights:

- When do I do it?
- What actions am I performing when I do it?
- What thoughts am I thinking?
- What emotions am I feeling?

If you catch yourself breath-holding, do not resume breathing by inhaling first. Instead, simply relax your entire body as you exhale out through your nose. Just take a moment to scan your body for any holding of tension, particularly through the neck, shoulders, upper back, chest, and abdomen. Let it all go, breathing in a relaxed and rhythmical way.

The chronic over-breather (hypocapnia)

If I asked you what would be better for you, to breathe more or breathe less, what would you respond? My guess is that, like most people, you would say that it would be better to breathe more. A common misconception is that by breathing in a larger volume of air we can increase the oxygen in our blood.

The amount of oxygen in your blood is called your oxygen

saturation (SpO_2), which is the percentage of hemoglobin molecules containing oxygen within the blood. A healthy individual would have an SpO_2 of around 97 to 98 percent. Because oxygen is constantly being diffused from the blood into the cells to create energy, having an SpO_2 of 100 percent may be a sign that oxygen delivery from your blood to your tissue isn't optimal, which is a typical sign that you are over-breathing.

Breathing in more than you need, to increase oxygen saturation in the blood, would be like continuing to refuel your car with gas even though the tank is already completely full—there is no functional purpose.

In fact, if you breathe in more than your metabolic demands require, rather than affect SpO_2 in any significant way, you are decreasing the concentration of arterial CO_2 in your blood, putting your body into a state called hypocapnia. Many people think of CO_2 as this toxic waste product that we need to get rid of, when actually it is the second most important gas in our blood after oxygen. If we didn't have carbon dioxide in our blood we would not be alive.

Chronic hypocapnia is a very serious problem, as the presence of carbon dioxide in our blood is critical for many vital functions in the body, including the delivery of oxygen to our cells (the Bohr effect).

Typical over-breathers will often breathe through the mouth at a faster rate, using secondary breathing muscles in the neck, shoulders, and chest. This is not to say that it's impossible to over-breathe when breathing diaphragmatically through the nose. In my experience, however, this is far rarer. There are many reasons why someone may develop an over-breathing habit, but the most common reason I see is chronic stress.

The controlled exhaler and aborted exhaler

The action of exhaling is as simple as relaxing all the muscles that worked to bring the air into your lungs on the inhale. The passive action of letting go allows the natural elastic recoil of these muscles to expel air. No extra energy is required.

As mentioned before, there are times when controlling the exhale is appropriate, for instance, when you're speaking, singing or exercising. The yogic Breathwork practice of pranayama includes many techniques that control the exhale, either speeding it up or slowing it down. There are many techniques in this book that use a controlled exhale for a designed physiological effect. But some people chronically and unconsciously control their exhale every moment of every day. I see this mostly in those who struggle to let go of control in other parts of their lives. These people often have type-A personality characteristics, are over-achievers, perfectionists, or struggle to delegate to others. Controlled exhaling is also more common with people who have lost trust in life because of a past hurt.

If you're trying to reduce anxiety and feel in control by controlling your exhale in this way, you're actually interrupting a natural process, rather than letting nature run its course. This can often result in one of two outcomes:

Pushing the exhale—breathing out more than needed. You're using extra effort and energy to control the exhale. Breathing out too much CO_2 can cause and shift your body into hypocapnia.

Aborting the exhale—interrupting the exhaling process before it is complete, with the next inhale. This can lead to feelings of breathlessness as CO_2 levels rise.

So, how are you supposed to breathe?

To help us define the characteristics of what optimal everyday breathing looks like, let's put together all the information we've looked at so far.

It's important to remember that your breathing will change depending on what you're doing, whether it's speaking, running, lifting, or swimming. That said, much of what we've been talking about is how to breathe when at rest. Establishing an optimal resting breath will serve you just as much as learning how to change your breath for different purposes, as described in the Breathwork techniques later in this book.

> ## OPTIMAL BREATHING . . .
>
> - Features inhaling and exhaling through the nose.
> - Uses a diaphragmatic breathing pattern (page 42).
> - Works at a speed that keeps your O_2 and CO_2 balanced—for most people around 10–14 breaths per minute.
> - Is rhythmical, with a natural pause in between the exhale and inhale.
> - Means relaxing and letting go of the exhale, no energy required.

Take the three breathing tests

Now you've learned a lot about the different ways to breathe, it's time to see how you breathe yourself! We're going to go through a series of tests to find out exactly how you breathe.

When I work one-to-one with clients, we go through a comprehensive series of tests and checks to assess the health and functionality of their breathing mechanics. We use technology and equipment to measure CO_2 and O_2 levels in the blood, heart rate variability, heart–brain coherence, and muscle tension and engagement (using surface electromyography). This is a lengthy and comprehensive process but what I'm providing here are three simple tests that you can do at home to easily assess the health of your own breathing. You'll only need three things:

- A way to film yourself (a smartphone is perfect).
- A way to time yourself (a stopwatch or smartphone).
- A tailor's measuring tape (or a piece of string you can measure later, after the test).

With these three things in hand, you're now ready to start the first test.

Test 1: Visual observation

Record yourself breathing. Watch yourself back. Identify your breathing pattern.

This test is used to determine which muscles you use to breathe. It's performed standing up. If you can, do this test without a top on, so you can see the movement of your body completely. Don't wear anything baggy, as you won't be able to see the movement of your body. Also, wearing anything too restrictive—tight clothes, belts, or jeans—may affect the way you breathe.

Record yourself breathing:

1. **Set up your phone/camera.** Or have someone hold it, so they're capturing your body from your head to your hips from a side-on view.

2. **Record yourself breathing for roughly 30 seconds.**
   Don't try to manipulate your breath in any way. Just
   relax and let the breath come and go as it pleases.
   Try to distract yourself by thinking about your last
   vacation or the recipe you used for the last meal that
   you made.

3. **After 30 seconds, take 3 slightly exaggerated
   breaths.** Inhale a little more than you usually would,
   just to emphasize which muscles you use to
   consciously breathe.

4. **Repeat the same steps.** Except this time from the
   front.

Can I do it in the mirror?

Yes, you can. However, the act of analyzing your
breath while you're breathing makes it far more likely
that you'll start to change the way you breathe.

Watch yourself back:

Once you've completed these steps, it's time to watch
yourself breathe. Don't worry about what you see. The
video may not look at all like what you were expecting.
Just observe and pay attention to the movement
of your:

- Neck and shoulders
- Upper chest, between your nipple line and your collar bones
- Mid and lower ribs, between your nipple line and your belly button
- Belly, between where your ribs end and your pubic bone

Identify your breathing pattern:

With these observations in mind, you can now classify your breathing pattern. Use the questions below to determine the assigned grade of your breathing pattern.

- As you inhale, does the movement begin in your upper chest?
- Do your shoulders rise?
- Does your chest aggressively puff out and upward?

If you said yes to these questions, your breathing is either chest breathing (grade C) or reverse breathing (grade D).

- Does your abdomen pull in toward the spine as you inhale?

If yes, your breathing is reverse breathing (grade D).

- As you inhale, does your abdomen remain still or does it only move minimally outward following your chest?

If yes, your breathing is chest breathing (grade C).

- Does the inhale initiate in your belly?
- Do your shoulders stay still?
- Does your chest remain still?
- Is there little to no sideways expansion in your mid to lower ribs?
- Does your abdomen forcefully expand forward and the sides of your abdomen pull inward?

If you said yes to these questions, your breathing is belly breathing (grade B).

- Does the inhale initiate in the diaphragm around the bottom of your ribs?
- Does your chest expansion follow the movement of your lower ribs?
- Do your shoulders stay still?
- Do your mid to lower ribs expand sideways?
- Does your abdomen expand passively following the movement of the ribs?

If you said yes to these questions your breathing is diaphragmatic breathing (grade A).

> ## When I watch myself breathe, I don't see any movement!
>
> For most people, their breathing at rest will be subtle, it won't be dramatic and big. In fact, chronically heavy breathing is a sign of dysfunction. However, if you see next to no movement at all, then you're most likely a no-breather (page 43). Consider this as a Grade C for this test.

Test 2: The vital capacity test

Measure after an exhale. Measure after an inhale. Grade your vital capacity.

Vital capacity (VC) is a common measure of the ability of your lungs to expand when you breathe. There are many factors that can decrease VC, including restrictive or obstructive lung diseases. Poor VC in healthy adults is primarily due to decrease in conditioning, attributable to aging or inactivity, lack of flexibility, and posture.

In the same way that tight hamstrings can prevent you from being able to touch your toes, the flexibility of the muscles around your spine and ribcage can have a big impact on your ability to expand your lungs. Even poor posture can affect the way you breathe. According to Dr. Rene Cailliet, a pioneer in the field of musculoskeletal medicine, poor posture can reduce lung capacity by as much as 30 percent.[3]

To do this test, you'll need a tailor's measuring tape or a piece of string.

Measure after an exhale (MAE):

1. **Wrap the tailor's measuring tape or piece of string around your chest.** Make it level with the very end of your sternum (the long flat bone running vertically down your chest in between your ribs) and running just beneath your shoulder blades.

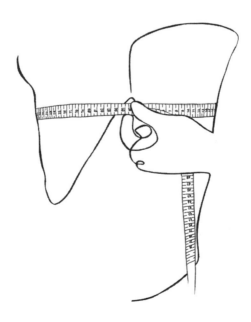

2. Take a deep breath in, then exhale completely. Empty your lungs as much as you can.

3. **Bring the measuring tape together, look down and take the reading.** Be sure to squeeze the tape around your chest firmly, but not so tightly that you create a false reading. If using a piece of string, pinch where the two ends of the string come together and then hold it against a normal ruler to take the reading.

Measure after an inhale (MAI):

1. **Wrap the tailor's measuring tape or piece of string around your chest.** Make it level with the very end of your sternum and running across your shoulder blades.

2. **Take a deep breath in, then exhale completely and take the deepest breath in that you can take.**

3. **Bring the measuring tape together, look down and take the reading.** Be sure to squeeze the tape around your chest firmly, but not so tightly that you create a false reading. If using a piece of string, pinch where the two ends of the string come together and then hold it against a normal ruler to take the reading.

Grade your VC:

Take the measurement after your inhale (MAI), then subtract the measurement after your exhale (MAE). This number is the change in the circumference of your ribcage.

Dividing this number by the measurement taken after your exhale (MAE) will give you a percentage. e.g. if your MAE is 73cm and your MAI is 81cm, your VC = (81–73)/73 = 0.109 or 10.9 percent.

- 10 percent or more—Grade A—Excellent VC
- 9–10 percent—Grade B—Good VC
- 8–9 percent—Grade C—Normal VC
- Below 8 percent—Grade D—VC needs improvement

Test 3: CO_2 tolerance test

Hold your breath and measure your time. Grade yourself.

This test is adapted from the Buteyko method (page 169) and uses a breath hold after an exhale to measure your physiological and psychological tolerance to a build-up of CO_2 in your blood.

When you hold your breath, it's the build-up of CO_2 in your blood that alerts you to breathe. A low tolerance to CO_2 is a great indicator of the possible presence of breathing pattern disorders, such as upper chest breathing and chronic over-breathing.

As people who are constantly anxious or experience panic attacks will often have a very low upper chest breathing tolerance to CO_2, it's also an indicator of your emotional reactivity or your ability to deal with stress.

An important note before we start. This test is not a measure of the maximum length of time that you can hold your breath. We will only hold our breath until we feel the first signs of "air hunger."

Safety notice:

Long breath-holding exercises should not be performed if you are pregnant or suffer from any of the following conditions:

- Epilepsy
- Uncontrolled blood pressure levels
- Sickle cell anemia
- Any severe heart problems in the past 6 months

If you are unsure whether this is safe for you, please consult your doctor.

Hold your breath and measure your time:

1. Start in a seated position and have your stopwatch ready.

2. Take a normal breath in through the nose, then exhale out normally through the nose. It's a relaxed exhale, so don't empty your lungs completely.

3. Pinch your nose with your fingers. This is to prevent sneaky inhales.

4. Start your stopwatch and count how many seconds until you feel the first indicators of air hunger. A good indicator is the involuntary movement of your muscles. Your belly may contract or twitch. Your neck and throat may contract.

5. Stop the stopwatch, release your nose, and take a breath in gently. If you feel like you need to take a big gasp of air, then you've held your breath for too long. You should be able to breathe normally and calmly right away.

Grade yourself:

Now that you have your number, it's time to grade yourself for this test.

- 10 seconds and under: **Grade D**
  - Your physical, mental and/or emotional health is likely being severely affected by your breathing. Breathing pattern disorders are almost certain and you're likely

feeling symptoms constantly, day to day (for
example, constant breathlessness or asthma
symptoms, feelings of unrest, anxiety, panic attacks).

- 10–20 seconds: **Grade C**
  - Your breathing is still not optimal. Symptoms as a
    result of breathing pattern disorders are likely
    experienced (for example, easy to become short of
    breath, inability to take a deep breath, constant
    blocked nose, asthma-like symptoms, easily anxious).
- 20–40 seconds: **Grade B**
  - Your breathing is likely adequate at rest. However, in
    certain situations (e.g., times of stress), your
    breathing is not serving you as well as it could.
- 40 seconds and more: **Grade A**
  - Your breathing is optimized to serve your physical
    health, mental performance, and emotional well-
    being—keep it up!

And that's it! You have completed your first breath
assessment. Hopefully, you now have three separate grades.

Three straight A's? Well done! Your breath is well optimized to
serve you.

If your three grades are either A or B, your breath is in a good
place, but there's still room for improvement.

C's or D's? You have some clear areas to work on.

Wherever you're currently at, it's time to enter your 21-day
Breathe Right program!

Our lungs are the planet's lungs

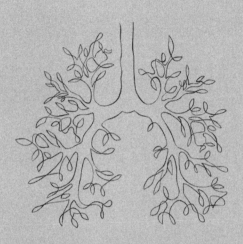

When we breathe in, our cells take in O_2 and produce CO_2, water, and energy. When trees, plants, and flowers breathe in, they do the exact opposite by taking in our exhaled CO_2, water, and energy (from the sun) to produce the O_2 that we will inhale with our next breath. Our respiratory system is not just inside us, but it is also all around us, intimately connected with nature. Our lungs even look like an upside-down tree!

3

THE 21-DAY *BREATHE RIGHT* PROGRAM

In this chapter, I'm going to introduce you to my 21-day *Breathe Right* program, which will help you kickstart your journey to optimizing your everyday breathing. It consists of a simple 20-minute daily practice, split up into two parts:

- **Core 15**—A 15-minute practice involving a series of stretches, muscle activation exercises, and breath-holding exercises; working to wake up your breathing system and optimize your breathing to serve you best. This remains the same for the entire 21 days.
- **Focus 5**—Five minutes of focused attention on the areas you need to improve most.

At the end of each week, you'll regrade yourself using the same three tests from the last chapter.
Each week you'll be able to adapt your Focus 5, based on which test you graded the lowest in. Let's begin with the Core 15.

The Core 15

Stretching

You might find that the muscles involved in your breathing movement can be stiff or tight. Often, these are the same muscles that become tight when we sit a lot or do lots of computer work. So, these stretches specifically target the muscles that directly and indirectly impact your breathing.

NOTE: There should never be pain when doing any of these stretches or exercises. If you feel pain, please back off the intensity of the stretch.

PEC TWISTS

This dynamic stretch uses movement to open up the front of the chest and mobilize your entire spine.

- Start in a standing position.
- Raise your left hand out at shoulder-height to your side, with your palm facing the sky.
- Put your right hand over your left pec.
- Twist toward your left as far as you can, until you feel some gentle resistance (you should feel a stretch in your back, your side, and your left pec).
- Freely twist with momentum back toward the center, as you extend your right arm out to your right side (palm facing up) and put your left hand over your right pec.
- Continue to twist back and forth, changing hands each time, until you have completed 10 on each side.

VERTICAL DOGS

This is a less strenuous version of the popular yoga posture—the "downward dog"—that everyone can do.

You'll be stretching your lats, a very large muscle that can impact flexibility of your thoracic cavity.

- Stand about two to three feet (depending on your size and flexibility level) away from a wall.

- With your arms straight, place your hands on the wall above your head with your palms facing inward.

- Start to lean into the wall, taking your head through your arms. Your arms should be quite straight but relaxed and not straining in any way. You should start to feel a stretch underneath your armpits and down your sides. Hold this stretch for 40 seconds.

FORWARD FOLD

Did you know that even the flexibility of your hamstrings can affect your breathing? It's time to stretch them out—as well as the rest of your posterior chain—with a basic forward fold.

- Start in a standing position with your feet hip-width apart.

- Take a deep breath in through your nose, then exhale through your mouth, as you bend forward at the hips, keeping your spine long until you feel a stretch in your hamstrings at which you can then relax your spine and let the crown of your head hang down loosely.

- Press your heels into the floor, as you lift up through your hips toward the ceiling. Make sure you keep a slight bend in your knees.

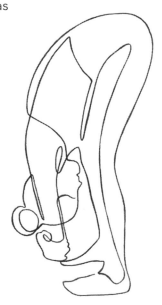

- You can either bend your elbows and hold on to each elbow with your opposite hand, or place your palms or fingertips on the floor beside your feet.

- As you hang, engage your quadriceps (the front thigh

muscles). The more you engage your quadriceps, the more your hamstrings will release.

- Hold the pose for up to 40 seconds, remembering to breathe gently all the way through.

- To release, place your hands on your hips. Inhale as you draw down through your tailbone; and keep your back flat as you rise up to standing position.

CAT–COW

This yoga classic involves movement back and forth between two poses that activate and stretch the back, abdominals, chest, and neck.

- Start on your hands and knees, with your wrists underneath your shoulders and your knees underneath your hips.

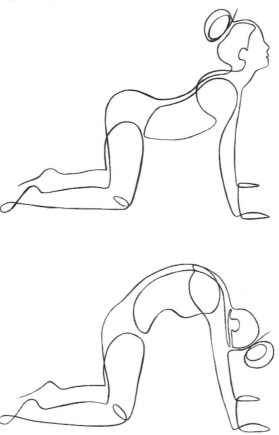

- Start with your spine in a neutral position, by extending forward through the crown of the head and back through the tailbone, keeping the neck long by looking down and slightly in front of you.
- Inhale and tilt your pelvis back, so that your tailbone sticks up.
- Your belly drops down, but keep your abdominal muscles engaged by drawing in toward your navel.
- Raise your gaze gently up toward the ceiling—only as far as you can go without cranking your neck.
- Hold this position for a couple of seconds.
- Exhale through your nose and tilt your pelvis forward, tucking in your tailbone and rounding your spine.
- Draw your navel toward your spine. Drop your head.
- Hold this position for a couple of seconds.
- Repeat 5 times.

GATE POSE

Known in yoga as Parīghāsana, this stretch is amazing for opening up the entire side of the torso from your neck to your hips. It may also stretch your hamstrings at the same time!

- Kneel on the floor. If this is painful for your knees, use a yoga mat, blanket, or cushion.

- If kneeling on the ground is not possible for you, you can perform the same stretch sitting on a chair, with both legs in front of your torso. Stretch one leg out to the side as demonstrated in the picture.

- Stretch your right leg out to the right and press your foot to the floor. Turn your right leg out, so that your kneecap is pointing toward the ceiling. This will require you to turn your hips slightly to the right, but not all the way.

- Make sure your left knee is directly aligned below your left hip.

- Reach your left arm up to the sky and slowly begin to bend over your right leg, allowing your right hand to slide down your thigh; stop once you feel a gentle stretch in your side.

- Stay in this pose for 30 seconds, before coming back up and repeating on the other side.

- Remember to breathe gently through your nose, lengthening a little more with each exhale.

PSOAS CONTRACT AND RELAX

The psoas is a deep-seated core muscle connecting the spine to the pelvic rim.

A tight psoas is a common culprit in lower back pain, sciatica, and other issues. However, as it is fascially attached to your diaphragm, it can also affect your breathing.

- Lie on your back with your arms by your side.
- Inhale through your nose and bring your knees to your chest. Curl yourself into a ball, trying to get your nose as close to your knees as possible (you can use your hands on your knees to pull your knees closer).
- Exhale through your mouth as you shoot your legs straight again and raise your arms above your head. Use some strength to lengthen your entire body as much as you can, then just relax into the floor for 2 seconds.
- Repeat 5 times.

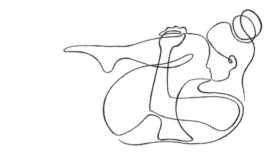

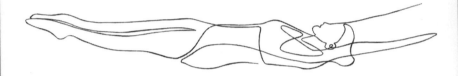

NOTE: If you have back pain or find this difficult to perform, you can do it one leg at a time. On the inhale, bring one leg toward your nose while leaving the other leg bent, with your foot on the floor. On the exhale, shoot both legs out to a straight position. Alternate legs.

SPINAL TWIST

Spinal twists are incredible for opening up your sides, stretching the diaphragm and intercostal muscles—as well as stimulating your abdominal organs by giving them a good squeeze!

- Lie on your back with your arms extended out to the side, like you're making the letter T.

- Bend your knees so the soles of your feet are on the floor, with your knees pointing toward the ceiling.

- Lift your hips off the floor and shift them a couple of inches off center to the right. This ensures that your hips are stacked vertically above each other and your spine is in a neutral position when you twist.

- Inhale and bring both your knees into your chest; as you exhale, slowly start to lower your knees to the left. Your right hip should be stacked (or as close to stacked as feels comfortable) over your left hip.

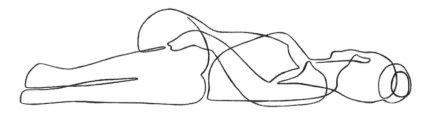

- Keep your right arm extended and look toward your right hand. You can rest your left hand on your right knee.

- Lie here for 1 minute, focusing on breathing slowly through your nose, relaxing into the stretch further with every exhale.

- After 1 minute, bring your knees back to center and place the soles of your feet back on the ground.

- Repeat for the other side, first lifting your hips off the floor, shifting them a few inches off center to the left.

NOTE: If your knees are very far from touching the ground, try putting pillows underneath your knees so they can relax.

SEATED SPINAL TWIST VARIATION

If you have back pain, are pregnant, or find this difficult to perform, you can do a variation while sitting on a chair.

- Sit sideways on a chair, pressing your left hip and thigh against the back of the chair. Make sure your hips, knees, and feet are all in line.

- Inhale and lift and lengthen up through the spine.

- Exhale and turn left to face the back of the chair and grab hold of the back of the chair with your right hand.

If you can, also press the palm of your left hand on the other side of the chair back.

- Hold this position for 1 minute, focusing on breathing slowly through your nose, relaxing into the stretch further with every exhale.

- After 1 minute, slowly come back to the center, releasing the chair. Change your position on the chair, so that your right hip and thigh are against the back of the chair.

- Repeat for the other side.

NOTE: As you twist, observe your knees. Has one moved forward? Focus on keeping the hips, knees, and feet squarely aligned.

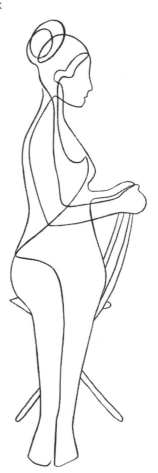

Now that we have stretched out many of the muscles in the body that support healthy breathing, we're going to target your breathing muscles directly. Let's begin with breathing see-saws—a fantastic exercise for warming up your primary breathing muscles.

WARMING UP YOUR BREATHING MUSCLES WITH BREATHING SEE-SAWS

There are two important concepts to grasp before doing this exercise: the idea of an ACTIVE action and the idea of a PASSIVE action.

When you're doing something ACTIVELY, you are consciously using your muscles and energy to make an action happen.

When you're doing something PASSIVELY, you're simply relaxing all your muscles and allowing the action to happen of its own accord.

As an example, if you lift your arm above your head, you are engaging the muscles in your arm and shoulder to ACTIVELY move your arm. If you then relax all the muscles in your arm and shoulder, your arm will PASSIVELY move as it flops back down to your side.

- Start in a lying position.
- ACTIVELY inhale through your nose, completely filling up your lungs.
- PASSIVELY exhale through your mouth, letting your lungs return to a neutral position.

- After a brief pause and without inhaling again, continue to ACTIVELY exhale through pursed lips, until you feel like you can't exhale any more, contracting the muscles in your ribs and abdomen.
- After a brief pause, relax all these muscles to PASSIVELY inhale, allowing fresh air to be sucked in through your nose, returning your lungs to a neutral position. There is no effort required to inhale, simply relax.
- Repeat this pattern 5 times.

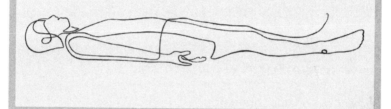

Now that we have warmed up your breathing muscles, it's time to focus on improving your breathing mechanics and CO_2 tolerance.

IMPROVING YOUR
BREATHING MECHANICS
AND CO_2 TOLERANCE

With this exercise, you accomplish two things. First, you improve your breathing mechanics. Second, you improve your CO_2 tolerance.

- Perform 20 breath cycles (explained below).
- Perform a breath hold (explained below).
- Repeat this pattern of breath cycle and breath hold 3 times in total.

How to perform a breath cycle

Depending on your grade for Test 1: Visual Observation, you'll use a different technique for the breath cycles. For both these techniques, you will breathe in and out through your nose.

IF YOU GRADED A OR B, PERFORM
DIAPHRAGMATIC BREATHING

In this technique, you'll focus on engaging the diaphragm completely. This is one breath cycle:

- Start in a lying position with knees bent and feet on the floor.
- Place your right hand over your navel and your left hand slightly above it (your pointer finger should be resting on the bottom of your sternum).
- Visualize where your diaphragm is and initiate the breath from this muscle.
- Inhale slowly and gently through your nose, breathing into your lower ribcage, making your ribcage expand in all directions. It might help to imagine breathing into your mid back. Inhale a little more air than you would on a normal breath, filling up your lungs by about 80 percent.
- You should feel your left (upper) hand move upward and sideways, while your right (lower) hand rises passively. However, don't force this movement. Keep your abdomen relaxed and let it move as a result of the downward movement of your diaphragm.
- Exhale through your nose and just relax, letting your ribcage and abdomen return to a neutral resting position.

As you get good at this breath, start to pay attention to other muscles in your body to see if you are engaging them in the breath.

Do your neck, shoulders, and shoulder blades move? Do any muscles in your face and jaw tense as you inhale or exhale?

Try to relax these as much as possible, until only your primary breathing muscles are being engaged.

IF YOU GRADED C OR D, PERFORM BELLY ISOLATION BREATHING

This is step one in learning how to breath diaphragmatically. The technique focuses on removing any unnecessary bracing or gut-sucking habits that you may have developed over time. This is one breath cycle:

- Start in a lying position with knees bent and feet on the floor.
- Place your right hand over your navel and your left hand on your chest.
- Inhale slowly and gently through your nose and focus on making your right (lower) hand rise while keeping the left (top) hand as still as possible.
- Don't feel like you need to fill up your lungs completely, as a deep breath will force you to

engage more muscles higher in your chest. Only inhale until just before your upper chest muscles begin to engage.
- Exhale through your nose and just relax, letting your abdomen return to a neutral resting position.

NOTE: For some people this will feel impossible. After all, you're trying to breathe in an opposite way to how you've breathed for many years.

If it feels very hard, don't get discouraged, it just takes patience and practice.

Keep experimenting, focusing on trying to engage different muscles.

Eventually, you'll get it!

How to perform breath-holding

This is performed in the same way as the breath-holding assessment outlined previously. Once you have completed your breath cycles, practice the steps below.

Remember, this test is not a measure of the maximum length of time that you can hold your breath. Here, we only hold our breath until we feel the first signs of air hunger.

You can time your breath holds if you want to. However, I encourage my clients to time their breath holds only when performing their assessments at the end of each week.

- Take a normal breath in through your nose and then exhale out normally through your nose (do not empty your lungs completely; it is a relaxed exhale).
- Pinch your nose with your fingers to prevent sneaky inhales.
- Just relax until you feel the first indicators of air hunger. A good indicator is the involuntary movements of your muscles. Your belly may contract or twitch. Your neck and throat may contract.
- Release your nose and take a gentle breath in. If you feel like you need to take a big gasp of air, then you have held your breath for too long. You should be able to breathe normally and calmly right away.

Safety notice:

Long breath-holding exercises should not be performed if you are pregnant or suffer from any of the following conditions:

- Epilepsy
- Uncontrolled blood pressure levels
- Sickle cell anemia
- Any severe heart problems in the past 6 months

If you are unsure whether this is safe for you, please consult your doctor.

Your Focus 5

Now that you've completed the Core 15, it's time to hone in on the primary area that you need to improve on.

So, looking at your grades for the three tests, pick the test with your lowest grade. Then follow the exercises below to improve that aspect of your breathing. If you have two or three tests with the lowest grade (e.g., two C's), alternate between them each day (or if you have time, do all of them!).

Visual test

If your visual test had the lowest grade, perform the following two exercises.

1. FOAM ROLLING

Soft foam rollers are so useful for increasing flexibility through the ribcage and thoracic spine. You can buy a soft foam roller online quite cheaply, and it can be used across many muscle groups in your body.

- Lie on your back with your legs bent and your feet on the floor.
- Place the foam roller in the middle of your back.
- Raise your arms above your head and interlock your fingers. Elbows are bent, arms are relaxed, letting gravity pull them toward the floor. Keep your butt grounded.

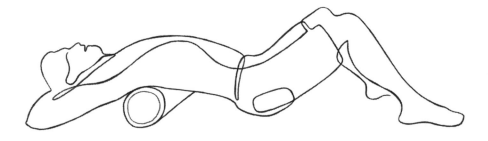

- You should feel pressure from the roller and a stretch through your lats, upper back, and ribcage, but no pain. If you feel pain, replace the foam roller with a rolled-up towel, which will act more gently on your back.

- Inhale through your nose into your lower/mid back for 4 seconds; then exhale through your nose or mouth (whichever feels best for you) for 4 seconds, relaxing further into the stretch.

- Stay here for 2 minutes. If you need a little break, you can hold the stretch for 45 seconds, rest for 30 seconds, then stretch again for 45 seconds.

2. WEIGHTED BELLY BREATHING

In this exercise, we'll use some extra weight placed on the belly to provide resistance and feedback for your belly breathing. You'll need a weight that can sit comfortably on your belly—a stack of books, a bag of rice, or even a kettlebell. Around 10 pounds will do nicely.

- Start in a lying position, with knees bent and your feet on the floor.

- Place your weight on your belly, just above your belly button.

- Inhale slowly through your nose and focus on pushing the weight on your belly toward the sky.

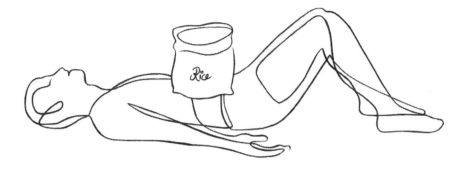

- Exhale and just relax, letting the abdomen return to a neutral resting position (this will feel quite quick, as there's extra weight on your belly).
- Repeat 30 times.

Vital capacity test

If your vital capacity test had the lowest grade, perform the following exercise.

1. FOAM ROLLING

Perform the same foam roller exercise as described in the visual test. Stay here for the full 5 minutes. If you need a little break, you can hold the stretch for 2 minutes, rest for 1 minute, then stretch again for 2 minutes.

CO_2 tolerance test

If your CO_2 tolerance test had the lowest grade, perform the following exercise.

1. THE DANCING DIOXIDE EXERCISE

If your grade was lowest in this test, let's get you doing an exercise to increase your tolerance to CO_2. The idea behind this exercise is to allow a tolerable level of CO_2 to accumulate in your blood. By breathing more slowly and with less volume, you keep CO_2 there for a longer period of time.

Safety notice:

This exercise should not be performed if you are pregnant or suffer from any of the following conditions:
- Epilepsy
- Uncontrolled blood pressure levels
- Sickle cell anemia
- Any severe heart problems in the past 6 months

If you are unsure whether this is safe for you, please consult your doctor.

- Start in a seated or lying position.
- Inhale slowly and gently, adopting either your diaphragmatic or belly isolation breathing pattern from pages 41–43 (you can place your hands on your chest and/or abdomen for guidance if you need it).
- Exhale and just relax, letting your abdomen return to a neutral resting position.
- Start to reduce the depth of your breath, making each inhale a little shorter than the last, until you feel a tolerable desire to breathe. Once you reach this point, maintain this depth of breath.
- This is where the exercise becomes like a dance. You will try to keep this air hunger consistent, either increasing it or decreasing it using your depth of breath. If it becomes too strong, increase the depth of the next few breaths slightly to bring CO_2 down to a tolerable level. If it becomes too easy, make the next inhale even shorter.
- If you feel like the urge to breathe has become too strong and that you need to gasp for air, then you've gone too far. If this happens, breathe normally for 15 seconds, then go back to reducing the depth of your breath.
- Over time, you will be able to significantly reduce the depth and movement of your breathing

muscles—it might even appear to you that you're not breathing at all!

- Also be aware of your emotions during this exercise—does it make you feel stressed or panicked, or can you relax into the slight discomfort you are experiencing?
- The goal of the exercise would be for you to maintain this tolerable desire to breathe for 5 minutes. But if you feel like you need to break it up into 30-, 45-, or 60-second rounds, that's totally fine.

Summary

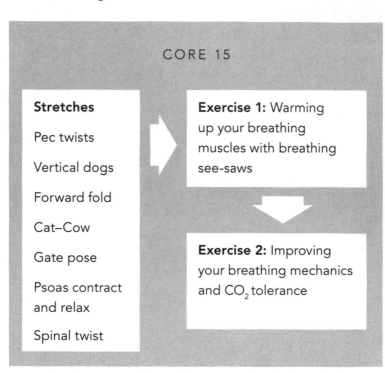

CORE 15

Stretches

Pec twists

Vertical dogs

Forward fold

Cat–Cow

Gate pose

Psoas contract
and relax

Spinal twist

Exercise 1: Warming
up your breathing
muscles with breathing
see-saws

Exercise 2: Improving
your breathing mechanics
and CO_2 tolerance

FOCUS 5

Visual test

Foam rolling

Weighted belly
breathing

**Vital capacity
test**

Foam rolling

**CO_2 tolerance
test**

Dancing dioxide

The way you breathe reflects how you feel

Think about the last time you felt stressed, anxious, or nervous. Did your breathing change? Perhaps you noticed that your breathing rate increased or that you started to breathe more shallowly. You may have even started to breathe in and out through your mouth. Maybe you found that you held your breath.

When we feel stressed, our bodies automatically change how we breathe. As a result, we usually breathe at a faster rate, using secondary breathing muscles in the upper chest that are not designed to be used all the time.

If you are constantly stressed, you will perform stressful breathing. When this occurs, not only has your breathing altered, but a whole host of changes are taking place simultaneously in your body without you even knowing.

The human body is a habit-forming machine. If you continue to breathe in this way, it becomes an unconscious habit. Even when an external stressor is gone, the breathing habit can remain. Then, just as the way you feel affects your breathing, the way you breathe affects the way you feel.

Continuing to breathe in this way over a prolonged period of time will start to result in adverse effects in your health. It may initially just feel like irritability, tension in your neck and shoulders, or difficulty sleeping.

It may then develop into anxiety, insomnia, chronic fatigue, digestive problems, and muscle pain, but it's not all doom and gloom. The good news is that the problem is also the solution. Because we can use our breath to change our physiology, we can also use it as a tool to manage our internal state.

4

YOUR DAILY BREATHWORK TOOL KIT

The rest of this book is dedicated to equipping you with the techniques you need to maximize this wonderful tool we call breathing.

Some of these techniques come from thousands of years of culture and tradition; others have been developed in the clinic, gym, or lab under strict research conditions. I've created many myself and tested them with clients, with hugely positive results. Regardless of a technique's origin, all we're doing is simply changing the way we breathe to affect our physiology and create a desired outcome.

In this chapter, we'll cover essential techniques that you can use on a daily basis, from the moment your eyes open in the morning until the time your head hits the pillow at night.

First, it's important to note that your relationship to your breath is unique to you, so breathing techniques will affect people differently. For example, some people find holding their breath after they've exhaled to be very stressful—not so great if the purpose of this technique is to try to relax!—while others find it blissfully peaceful.

What I'm offering is simply a guide with lots of options and variations—the most important thing is that you follow how you feel. These techniques are an invitation to become aware of your physical, mental, and emotional state. Observing your breath and how it affects you is one of the most intimate forms of introspection that you can do.

Tip:

When you're first learning breathing techniques, you'll often be encouraged to focus on the length of each part of the breath (e.g. inhale for 3 seconds, exhale for 6 seconds). However, it's just as important to emphasize which muscles you're using to breathe in and out. So, throughout all the upcoming techniques, I'd like you to assume that every breath you take is using correct diaphragmatic breathing, as outlined in the previous chapter, unless I tell you otherwise.

Get used to the breath volume (BV) scale

There are many characteristics of the breath that you can alter to make up a breathing technique. One of the characteristics that often gets lost when teaching a technique is the volume of the inhale and exhale, which can have a big effect on the end result. In the following exercises I will be emphasizing the volume of the inhale and exhale—using a breath volume (BV) scale that goes from 1 to 10 as an indicator as to how much volume you should breathe in or out. To get a feel for this scale, perform the following:

- Take a complete breath in, filling your lungs completely. You should feel expansion in your belly, chest, and clavicular (around your collar bone) areas. That's BV 10.
- Exhale without force, as you relax every muscle in your body, until your chest and abdomen have shrunk back to their neutral size. This is BV 5.
- Now use some energy to exhale out with vigor, squeezing your abdominals until you feel like you have no more air left in your lungs. This is BV 1.

The first step of Breathwork: breath awareness

The first and most important step of any Breathwork practice is simply to draw your attention to your breath without changing its behavior. You are the observer, the watcher, and the witness of nature in action. Your breath is the anchor to the here and now; it's never in the past, never in the future.

It just so happens that this practice by itself is very relaxing, even if a little challenging at first. It can be very hard to observe your breath and not take control of it, particularly for people who struggle to let go of control in one or many aspects of their life.

The way we breathe is such a reflection of how we approach life. So, for someone who likes to be in control all the time, letting the breath happen without taking charge of it may be a challenge. But, with practice, it will become easier and you'll be able to allow your breath to come and go reflexively without you getting in the way.

PRACTICE BREATH AWARENESS

- Sit comfortably.
- Close your mouth and allow the breath to come and go through the nose.
- Start by noticing the physical sensations of breathing:
  - Track the flow of air through your nose into your lungs—what does it feel like?
  - Which muscles move as you breathe?
- Next, start to pay attention to the natural reflexes of your breathing:
  - When does your body want to inhale and for how long?
  - Does your body want to pause at the top of the inhale?
  - When does your body want to start to exhale and for how long?
  - Does your body want to pause at the bottom of the exhale?
- Continue to observe the breath in its reflexive form. There's no right or wrong, nothing to achieve,

nothing to get right. Simply observe with curiosity. Let the breath breathe you!

- For its relaxing effect, repeat for at least 3–5 minutes. This practice is fantastic for meditation, so you can keep going for as long as you want.

It's completely normal for your mind to wander off or become distracted during this practice, no problem! Once you realize that you've gone off tangent, simply bring your awareness and focus back to the next breath.

Now for some suggestions on how to use your breath for different parts of your day!

MORNING MOTIVATOR

BREATHING TO WAKE UP THE BODY

Start your day with some big breath surfing

When we're asleep, many of our vital functions drop, including our respiratory rate, heart rate, and blood pressure. So leaping out of bed as soon as we wake up may not be the best idea. As your body tries to adapt to this sudden action, this can lead to undue stress.

Instead, you can use your breath to gently wake up your body and stimulate your respiratory, nervous, cardiovascular, lymphatic, and digestive systems into higher action.

The reason I call this exercise "big breath surfing" is that in it, we use our breath to create a wave of movement through our body. Starting in our belly, coming up through the midribs, and finishing up in the chest—we are literally surfing the waves of our breath. It certainly beats lying in bed scrolling through social media feeds on your phone for 10 minutes!

BIG BREATH SURFING

- While lying in bed, put one hand over your belly button and one hand on your chest, with the fingertip of your index finger touching the bottom of your sternum (so your hand is on the side of your ribs).
- Breathe through your nose into your belly, making your belly hand rise by an inch or two, barely moving the hand on your sternum (BV 7).
- Exhale out through the mouth with a relaxed sigh (BV 5).
- Repeat this pattern 3 times.
- Next, breathe through your nose, first making your belly hand rise. One second after the belly hand has started to rise, allow your breath to start coming up into your midribs, feeling them expand sideways (BV 8).
- Exhale out through your mouth with a relaxed sigh (BV 5).
- Repeat this pattern 3 times.
- Next, repeat the belly and midribs breath, but, this time, soon after the midribs have started to expand, allow your breath to come all the way up to your collar bones (BV 9).
- Exhale through the mouth with a relaxed sigh (BV 5).
- Repeat this pattern 3 times.

AFTERNOON BOOSTERS

BREATHING FOR ENERGY

Breath of fire
(Kapalbhati pranayama)

Originating from the yogic breathing practice of pranayama, this exercise is designed to bring clarity to the frontal region of your brain—which is responsible for higher-order brain functions, such as advanced cognition, sensory perception, initiation of motor commands, and language. The kind of functions you're going to need on the early afternoon shift!

The important thing to note about performing Kapalbhati is that your energy is focused on the exhale, while the inhale is passive. Since you've put force into the exhale, air will be automatically drawn in on the inhale as soon as you relax. You effectively do the exhale, then let the inhale do itself. I've added an extra breath step to the traditional Kapalbhati, which my clients and I really enjoy.

Safety notice: If you are pregnant or suffer from any stomach issues (for example, stomach ulcers), you should not perform this exercise.

- This breath can be done seated or standing.
- Exhale forcefully through your nose, also with a forceful contraction of your abdominal muscles (BV 3).
- Following the exhale, allow the inhalation to happen by itself as you relax your abdominal muscles (BV 5).
- Complete 20 rapid breaths.
- Inhale through your nose completely (BV 9).
- Hold your breath for 10 seconds.
- While holding your breath, relax your abdomen, back, chest, shoulders, and neck—you may feel some slight pressure go into your head.
- Sigh out through your mouth and relax for a few seconds (BV 5).
- Repeat this 3 times.

The Energizer Bunny

Next time you're itching for that late afternoon coffee, save yourself the money and just breathe, it's free! The Energizer Bunny is a variation of a technique from the Sufi tradition. I call it this because, in the breath, you'll be sniffing through your nose quickly, which often makes people twitch their nose, just like a little rabbit!

The pace of the breath is fast and fills your lungs completely. This combination of fast pace and deep breathing is incredibly stimulating and very helpful if you're feeling sleepy or groggy and need a quick boost of energy.

This breath may make you start to feel a little light-headed and you may even experience some buzzing sensations in your body. This is all completely normal, so don't stress. Everything returns to normal within a matter of seconds of finishing the breathing, except that you'll now feel far more energized!

- This breath can be done seated or standing.
- Exhale in a relaxed manner (BV 5).
- Take three quick and powerful inhales through your nose, progressively filling up your lungs more and more. The length of the inhales are equal. On your final inhale, your breath volume should be up to BV 9.
- Exhale with a big sigh through your mouth (BV 5).
- That completes one breath cycle. Aim to complete 36 breath cycles per minute, so each breath takes a little under 2 seconds to complete.
- Repeat this pattern for 45–60 seconds and notice the difference in how you feel!

STRESS BUSTERS

BREATHING FOR RELAXATION

In 2018, a UK-wide survey on stress showed that 74 percent of the participants had at some point over the past year felt overwhelmed or unable to cope with a situation as a result of stress.[4]

The physiological response of stress is governed by the autonomic nervous system (ANS). The ANS is the part of your nervous system that regulates the vital automatic and involuntary processes such as your heart rate, blood pressure, breathing, and digestion.

The ANS is split into two components, the sympathetic nervous system (SNS) and the parasympathetic nervous system (PNS). Think of the SNS as the gas pedal for our body. It triggers the "fight or flight" (and lesser known "freeze") response, mobilizing the body to be ready for action so that it can respond to a perceived danger. Once the danger has passed, the PNS provides the brake and promotes the "rest and digest" response that in turn promotes relaxation and restoration in the body. If your SNS is the gas pedal and your PNS is the brake, consider your breath to be the driver in charge!

Coherent breathing

When we feel relaxed, we are experiencing higher activity in our PNS. The level of activity in the PNS is reflected in your heart rate variability (HRV), a measure of the natural variations of time between your heartbeats.

Many people would say having less variation in the time between heartbeats (a low HRV) is desirable, when actually a healthy variation of time between heartbeats (a higher HRV) is an indicator of a balanced and flexible nervous system and a healthy cardiovascular system. One of the most effective ways to influence your HRV is by your breathing.

First described in Stephen Elliot's book *The New Science of Breath*, coherent breathing is breathing at a rate of 5 breaths per minute (6-second inhale, 6-second exhale) and has been shown to optimize HRV.[5]

- Start in a seated or lying position.
- Inhale through your nose for 6 seconds (BV 8).
- Exhale through your nose for 6 seconds (BV 3).
- Repeat this cycle for at least 3 minutes, but there really is no limit as to how long you can go.
- If 6 seconds feels like a struggle, reduce it to 5 or 4 seconds and get comfortable breathing at that rate first. You can then gradually build it up to 6 seconds.
- If you are over 6 feet tall, you may want to breathe even slower: try 7 seconds in and 7 seconds out.
- For children under the age of 10, try 4 seconds in and 4 seconds out.

Try this

Find your pulse on your wrist and then start to slow down your breathing, inhaling for 4 seconds and exhaling for 4 seconds. Pay attention to the speed of your pulse when you inhale versus when you exhale. Did you notice that your pulse slows down as you exhale? So you can see that the variability of your heart rate is quickly influenced by the way that you breathe.

5pm breathing

In this technique, you'll exhale for longer than you inhale and pause briefly after the exhale. Studies have shown that by extending the exhale to be longer than your inhale, you can significantly increase the level of activity in your vagus nerve, the longest nerve of the ANS, which in turn will activate your relaxation response.[6]

I call this technique 5pm breathing because 5 p.m. is supposed to be that joyous moment where some of us get to knock off work, relax, and let our hair down. It also stands for 5 breaths per minute and is designed to help you wind down and de-stress your internal systems.

- Start in a seated or lying position.
- Inhale for 4 seconds through your nose (BV 8).
- Exhale for 6 seconds through your nose (BV 3).
- Hold your breath for 2 seconds.
- That's one breath cycle.
- Repeat this breath cycle at least 10 times.
- You can keep repeating it until you have reached your desired state of relaxation.

Twice the Calm breathing

If holding your breath after the exhale in 5pm breathing felt uncomfortable, then try this breathing technique. It is called Twice the Calm because we're doubling the length of the part of the breath that activates the vagus nerve—the exhale.

- Start in a seated or lying position.
- Inhale for 4 seconds through your nose (BV 8).
- Exhale for 8 seconds through pursed lips (BV 3).
- That's one breath cycle.

Repeat this breath cycle at least 15 times, or you can keep repeating it until you've reached your desired state of relaxation.

- If 8 seconds feels like too long, go to 3–6 or 2–4 and slowly work your way up until 8 seconds is comfortable.

Bumble bee breath
(bhramari pranayama)

This is another classic from the yogic breathing practice of pranayama that's been shown to decrease the heart rate and also blood pressure.[7] This technique requires you to make some noise, so it may not be the best one to use in a quiet office, but it's excellent to use at home or on a noisy bus or train.

- Sit comfortably with your back straight.
- Close your mouth and lips.
- Inhale slowly through your nose (BV 8).
- Exhale through your nose while making a "mmm" humming sound, just like the buzzing of a bee (BV 3).
- The sound should be soft, but loud enough so that you feel the front of your face and skull vibrate.
- You can even experiment humming at different pitches, to see if it has a different effect.
- Repeat at least 5 times or as many times as you need to feel the effect.
- For the full effect, you can even use your index fingers to block your ears by pushing down on the flap (tragus) just outside where your ear canal begins. This enhances the effect of the sound as you hum.

EVENING CALMERS

BREATHING FOR SLEEP

In Dr. Matthew Walker's book, *Why We Sleep*, he states that "the leading causes of disease and death in developed nations—diseases that are crippling health-care systems, such as heart disease, obesity, dementia, diabetes, and cancer—all have recognized causal links to a lack of sleep."

So, how can our breathing help us get some better shut-eye? The body is excellent at developing habits. If you're in action mode all day, every day, your physical systems will be very good at staying in that mode. This means that, even once your head hits the pillow, your body isn't going to make it easy for you to switch off, no matter how comfortable your bed. However, you can use your breathing to calm your nervous system down, teaching it to shift from a state of high arousal to a state of rest and relaxation. Focusing on your breath will also help you to come into the present moment and slow down those racing thoughts.

Here is a selection of techniques that have really helped my clients to catch more z's. So, next time you're tossing and turning in bed, I would suggest giving these a try.

Ladder breathing

In this breath, you progressively increase the length of your inhales and exhales, concentrating on what it feels like to change the rhythm of your breathing as your nervous system is slowly calmed.

This slow breathing promotes parasympathetic activity, while the change in counts keeps the mind occupied.

- To be performed while lying in bed.
- Inhale slowly through your nose for a count of 4 seconds (BV 8).
- Exhale slowly through your nose for a count of 4 seconds (BV 3).
- Next, inhale for a count of 5 seconds, then exhale for a count of 5 seconds.
- Keep increasing the length of your inhales and exhales until you get to 10 seconds in and 10 seconds out.

NOTE: There is no need to push to 10 seconds if it doesn't feel comfortable. Only extend your breathing as far as feels easy for you.

- Once you reach 10 seconds, you can either continue to breathe at this pace, keep increasing the length of your inhales and exhales, or even go up and down the ladder.
- If you choose to come back down, I wouldn't go back any lower than 6 seconds per inhale and exhale.

Breathe and release

Breathe and release is a variation of progressive muscle relaxation, a relaxation therapy in which you systematically contract and then relax each muscle group in your body. This technique combined with the breath provides a powerful formula for relaxing physical tension in the body and relaxing your mind at the same time.

- To be performed while lying in bed.
- Slowly inhale through your nose (the exact length isn't important, as long as it's slow).
- As you inhale, imagine you're breathing into a specific muscle group; and, as you breathe into it, slowly tense that muscle more and more, until you've reached the top of your inhale.
- It may take a little bit of practice to coordinate the breath and muscle tension at the same time.
- Hold your breath and the tension for a couple of seconds.
- As slowly as you can, start to exhale through the nose; as you exhale, slowly relax the tensed muscle group until it feels like it's jelly.
- Repeat this process for all the muscle groups in your body, starting with your forehead and working all the way down to your toes.

4–7–8 breathing

4–7–8 breathing was made popular by celebrity doctor Dr. Andrew Weil. This technique originates from pranayama and acts as "a natural tranquilizer for the nervous system" that eases the body into a state of calmness and relaxation. The anecdotal evidence is outstanding. To get the most out of this technique, Dr. Weil suggests that you should practice this technique at least twice a day as well as when you want to sleep. After a couple of weeks of daily practice, one of my students found this technique so effective that he would rarely get to the final cycle of breath before he fell asleep.

- To be performed while lying in bed.
- First, place the tip of your tongue against the ridge of tissue just behind your upper front teeth, and keep it there through the duration of the exercise.
- You will be exhaling through your mouth around your tongue; if this seems awkward, try pursing your lips slightly.
- Exhale through your mouth—you'll make a soft whoosh sound (BV 2). It may feel a little strange exhaling around your tongue so practice it a few times to get used to it.

- Close your mouth and inhale gently through your nose for 4 seconds (BV 8).
- Hold your breath for 7 seconds.
- Exhale through your mouth with some force, making a soft whoosh sound for 8 seconds (BV 3).
- This completes one breath cycle.
- Repeat the cycle 3 more times for a total of 4 breath cycles. If you feel comfortable doing this you can increase the number of cycles to 8, but never more than that.
- NOTE: If this breath feels very slow, you can count a little faster than a standard second and slow it down over time. The most important thing is that you keep the ratio of inhale–hold–exhale as 4 counts–7 counts–8 counts.

Breathing for chronic lower back pain

Multiple studies have found correlation between lower back pain and breathing pattern disorders. Physical therapists and other health practitioners around the world are now placing greater emphasis on correct breathing as a path of treatment for patients with lower back pain.

Some of the primary and secondary muscles used for breathing are connected to the lumbar spine and are also key stabilizer muscles. When these are not functioning correctly, it can cause havoc with your lower back.

By following the 21-day *Breathe Right* program (Chapter 3), you will make big strides in retraining your breathing mechanics back to their optimal state. However, sometimes back pain isn't just about the mechanical structures of your body.

Dr. John Sarno, a world-famous back pain specialist, believed that much back pain was actually a symptom of a psychosomatic process stemming from emotional factors. In his book *The Divided Mind: The Epidemic of Mindbody Disorders*, he explained that the brain distracts by making us feel pain to stop us experiencing negative emotions.

For example, rather than acknowledging that we are in a toxic relationship, hate our job, or haven't dealt with past traumas, the brain will make us focus on pain.

Sarno believed that pain was created by the brain unconsciously reducing blood flow, and therefore oxygen, to the muscles and nerves of the back.

In my work, I have seen many clients who have previously tried all sorts of physical treatments to no avail, before having success with Breathwork. On occasion, I've witnessed an instant and permanent remission of symptoms.

See page 193 to learn more about Integrative Breathwork, a method that can be useful in these instances.

5

A WORLD OF BREATHING TECHNIQUES

Now that we have covered techniques that everyone will find useful, the rest of this book is dedicated to providing techniques for specific situations in your life. Not all of them may be relevant to you now, but keep this book in mind, as you never know which techniques may be useful to you in the future. I've split the final chapter into five sections:

Mental well-being—anger and frustration; road rage; nervousness; anxiety and panic attacks; performance anxiety; mental rehearsal; decision-making; creativity; focus and concentration; meditation.

Sports performance—nasal breathing benefits; high-altitude training; post-workout recovery.

Physical health—better sex; quitting smoking; headaches and migraines; asthma; high blood pressure; pain; hangovers; nausea and motion sickness.

The Wim Hof Method—autoimmune diseases; endometriosis; chronic pain and fatigue; irritable bowel syndrome; altitude sickness.

Integrative Breathwork—the extraordinary healing power of the breath.

MENTAL WELL-BEING

Anger and frustration

Have you ever considered why you sigh? Usually you don't do it on purpose; it just happens.

Researchers from the University of Leuven suggest that sighing acts as a physical, mental, and emotional reset. In one study, the researchers observed the breathing patterns of participants for 20 minutes while sitting quietly and noticed that the nature of the way they breathed, such as volume and speed, was different before and after a sigh.[8] When your breathing pattern remains constant and unchanged for an extended period of time (such as fast and shallow when you are stressed or anxious), your lungs become stiffer, leading to less efficient gas exchange.

A sigh is a break in your constant pattern of breathing to reset your respiratory system. Defined as an inhale that's twice as large as normal, it stretches the alveoli (the air sacs in your lungs), giving you a sense of comfort and relief. Hence, the common term, "a sigh of relief."

Breathwork master Dan Brulé, author of *Just Breathe*, was the first person to open my mind to the idea of using a "sigh of relief" on purpose. If we already have a natural reflex built into us that helps us reset, then why don't we use it on purpose!

- Start in a seated, standing, or lying position.
- Slowly inhale through your nose (BV 9), expanding your abdomen and your chest.
- Once you get to the top of your inhale, sigh out through the mouth (BV 5), without pause. No effort or control is required. This bigger-than-normal inhale will mean that, as soon as you relax all your breathing muscles and open your mouth, the exhale will naturally escape out of you with gusto. Really let go of the breath and let it fall out of you.
- Use it as an opportunity to let go of other things. Let go of your muscles, let go of your joints, let go of your worries or thoughts that are making you angry.
- Repeat 10 times or as many times as required.

Experiment with different exhale sounds

When exhaling, you can experiment with different mouth shapes to see which brings you the most pleasure. For example, a "Haaaaaa" sigh may feel different to a "Pooooooo" sigh, which may in turn feel different to a "Shhhhhhhhh" sigh.

Road rage

In the car, you can do things that aren't that appropriate to do in public, like making a lot of sound!

In this technique, you'll make an "Aahh" sound on the exhale. Sounding and chanting can be found in many ancient traditions, such as Tibetan Buddhism, Hinduism, Native American tradition, and Sufism, and new research is showing how it can affect the brain positively. A study published in the *International Journal of Yoga* found that chanting reduced activity in the parts of the brain responsible for emotion and controlling the stress response.[9] At the end of the day, being able to sound out your anger and frustration always feels good.

- Inhale through the nose (BV 9) for a count of 4.
- Exhale through the mouth and sound "Aahh" at a loud volume for as long as you can.
- Really squeeze out as much air as you can, without straining your throat.
- Repeat 5 times.
- If you feel as though the "Aahh" sound wants to change into a different sound, maybe try an "Eeehhh" or even an "Ooommm" sound—let it change!
- Once complete, perform a few sighs of relief (page 129), then just relax and breathe through your nose again, slowly.

NOTE: Please concentrate on the road when performing this technique!

Feeling nervous

Here's a technique used by Navy SEALS to calm their nerves before going into combat. If it is good enough for the SEALS before entering a life or death situation, then it's good enough for me! Not only does this breath help to relax your nervous system, its balanced pattern helps to instill a feeling of being in control.

It's called box breathing. The breath is broken down into four equal parts, like the sides of a square. The length of each part should be whatever feels comfortable to you.

- This can be done seated, standing, or lying.
- Exhale through your nose (BV 5).
- Inhale through your nose slowly for a count of 5 seconds (BV 8). Remember your diaphragmatic breathing!
- Hold your breath for a count of 5.
- Use this breath hold as a good chance to scan your body for any tension and release it.
- Exhale slowly through your nose for a count of 5 (BV 3).
- Hold your breath for a count of 5.
- Again, focus on releasing any tension held in your body.
- Repeat this pattern of inhale—pause—exhale—pause for at least 3 minutes, or until you have felt yourself fully calm down.

Eventually, this breathing pattern will be such an anchor for relaxation for you that you may only have to do it once or twice for your nerves to disappear. While a good place to start is 4 or 5 seconds, you could make the lengths even longer if you like.

Anxiety and panic attacks

When I work with clients who struggle with anxiety or panic attacks, I create little breathing rituals they can do when they feel a panic attack coming on and when they're in the middle of one.

While each ritual is tailored to the individual, here's one example that I find works very well for many people. As the breath calms down your nervous system, mindfully rubbing your hands together has been shown to generate delta waves in the brain, which in turn prompt helpful chemical chain reactions in the amygdala, the fear center of the brain.

- First, you must gain control over your breath and begin to slow it down. Put one hand on your belly to make sure that you're breathing diaphragmatically. Also make sure your shoulders and neck are relaxed and not holding tension.
  - Inhale through your nose for 3 seconds (BV 8) and exhale for 3 seconds (BV 3).
  - Repeat.
  - Inhale through your nose for 4 seconds (BV 8) and exhale for 4 seconds (BV 3).
  - Repeat.
  - Inhale through your nose for 5 (BV 8) seconds and exhale for 5 seconds (BV 3).
- Now give yourself a big sigh of relief (page 129).
- After the exhale from the sigh, pause your breathing for around 10 seconds. Notice the stillness that can be experienced in the pause between two breaths, knowing that the next inhale is just around the corner.
- While holding your breath, repeat the following sentence in your head, "What I'm feeling is my body preparing for action. It's a natural response of self-love and protection. It will soon pass."
- Now give yourself another big sigh of relief.
- Begin to perform the Twice the Calm breath exercise (page 114).

- After a few cycles of performing Twice the Calm breath, continue this pattern as you start rubbing the palms of your hands together and focus on the warmth being generated between your hands.
- Continue this combination of breathing and rubbing your hands for at least 3 minutes, or as long as you like.

Feel free to tweak the ritual with any of the other techniques that you find useful in this book, or even make up your own!

Performance anxiety/stage fright/ fear of public speaking

Whether you are an Olympic athlete about to perform on the big stage or a student about to go into an important exam, the anxiety and fear before a performance can be crippling.

In these situations, I like to add a couple of extra steps before the previously mentioned box breathing technique (page 133) to create a powerful routine to take you out of those paralyzing states of nervousness. I call this routine "Stepping down," which will focus on three things: 1) pausing and focusing on relaxing your body; 2) balancing your blood gas levels, as you'll almost certainly have been hyper-ventilating; 3) continuing to calm down your nervous system.

- Start in a comfortable standing or seated position.
- Perform 7 sighs of relief (page 129). On each exhale, focus on relaxing a single body part, starting from the top to the bottom, beginning with:
    - Exhale 1—Forehead
    - Exhale 2—Eyebrows
    - Exhale 3—Eyes
    - Exhale 4—Cheeks
    - Exhale 5—Mouth
    - Exhale 6—Jaw
    - Exhale 7—Neck
- After the 7th exhale, hold your breath. The purpose of this breath hold is not to hold your breath for as long as possible. Only hold your breath for as long as feels comfortable.
- During this breath hold, repeat to yourself, "This feeling I am having is my body's way of preparing me for action. I am ready."
- Perform 5 sighs of relief. On each exhale, focus on relaxing a single body part. Continuing down the body:
    - Exhale 1—Shoulders
    - Exhale 2—Arms
    - Exhale 3—Hands
    - Exhale 4—Chest and upper back
    - Exhale 5—Abs and lower back

- After the 5th exhale, hold your breath again for as long as feels comfortable. During this breath hold, repeat the mantra on the previous page.
- Perform 3 sighs of relief. On each exhale, focus on relaxing a single body part. Continuing down the body:
  - Exhale 1—Thighs
  - Exhale 2—Calves
  - Exhale 3—Feet and toes
- After the 3rd exhale, hold your breath again for as long as feels comfortable. During this breath hold, repeat the mantra.

Begin box breathing (page 133) for as long as feels right for you.

Melanie was an aspiring young opera singer in her final years of her music education at a conservatorium of music. While blessed with an incredible voice, her biggest struggle when performing was her uncontrollable nerves, causing her to feel out of breath and her throat to tense up. This was a big deal for her, as it meant she wasn't able to comfortably hit the top of her vocal range. Just knowing this gave her more anxiety and caused her to become even more tense. In our first session I taught her the stepping down routine. She practiced it for 5 minutes every day for a week so that the sequence became easy and natural and she didn't have to think about it. Before her next performance exam, she started to use the step down 5 minutes before she was assessed. She felt calm and in a state of flow as she performed her piece perfectly, even reaching the highest notes with ease.

Mental rehearsal

Whether you're an athlete, musician, or performer of any kind, visualization of a successful performance before you have to do it has been shown to be a powerful tool to enhance your performance.

Research has shown that slowly inhaling through the nose has an effect on the emotional and memory centers of the brain, which can lead to better memory and recall.[10] Couple this with a slow exhale to shift you into your rest and relaxation mode (the optimal state to learn in) and you have a powerful hack for your visualization practice.

- Start seated, standing, or lying in a comfortable position.
- Inhale through your nose slowly for a count of 5 seconds (BV 8).
- As you inhale, visualize the steps, moves, or moments that you need to execute.
- Exhale slowly through your nose for a count of 5 (BV 3).
- As you exhale, relax your mind, only focusing on your breath.
- Repeat this pattern of inhales and exhales until you have reached the end of your performance/ execution.
- Once complete, perform 3 sighs of relief (page 129). With each sigh, try to imagine the feeling of satisfaction, joy, and accomplishment of successfully completing your performance. Enjoy the moment, you did it!

Decision-making

You can call it your intuition, unconscious, or gut feeling, but I believe the body has an innate wisdom that knows the truth and what's best for you. But many of us have become so disconnected from this wisdom. There are many therapies, such as kinesiology, that use somatic tests and cues to access this wisdom. You can even do it with your breath!

This technique provides you with a tool to access this wisdom and help you make decisions about your day and your life. If you have a question or a decision to make, use your breath to tap into this wisdom and see if it can provide you with guidance.

To build up the sensitivity of your awareness of how your breath makes you feel, you can perform the following exercise:

Feeling the "Yes" breath:

- First, take a few slow coherent breaths (page 112) to bring your awareness to your breath.
- Exhale through your nose (BV 5). This is important because you still need enough air to say a statement out loud.

- Now, out loud, say an obviously true statement (e.g., "My name is Richie.").
- Now, inhale through the nose (BV 8) and just notice how that breath feels.
- Sigh in a relaxed way out through the mouth (BV 5).
- That's the first breath done. Take a moment, breathing normally, to reflect on how it made you feel.

Feeling the "No" breath:

- When you're ready, exhale through the nose (BV 5).
- Now, out loud, say an obviously false statement (e.g., "My name is John.").
- Now, inhale through the nose (BV 8) and just notice how that breath feels.
- Sigh in a relaxed way out through your mouth (BV 5).

Can you feel the difference in the breath? When doing the breath after the obviously false statement, maybe there's some tightness in the throat or more resistance as you breathe. Maybe your shoulders rise or your jaw clenches a little.

Go back and forth and try different true/false statements so that you can start to tell a difference between a "Yes" and "No" breath. While it may take a little practice, it's so useful once you get the hang of it.

Once you can start to tell the difference, use it to make decisions:

- First, create a positively framed statement, then say it out loud and then take a breath to see if it agrees with you. It's important to frame the statement in the positive (e.g., "I am, I will") instead of the negative (e.g., "I won't, I shouldn't"). Some examples of statements could be:
  - "I will enter into a business partnership with this person."
  - "I will take this university course."
  - "I am in a happy and healthy relationship."

Creativity

Being creative means taking a break from habitual and automatic thinking to come up with new and outside-of-the-box ideas. In other words, the human brain must ignore the most obvious and common ideas to reach new and creative ones. Recent research has found that this process is optimized to occur when higher levels of alpha brainwaves are present, particularly in the right hemisphere of the brain (responsible for imagination, creativity, insight, visuospatial material, and music).[11]

For this technique, we will combine either Energizer Bunny (page 109) or Breath of Fire (page 107) to create some energy and alertness with probably the most famous technique coming out of pranayama, alternate nostril breathing (nadi shodhana). It is famously publicized that Hillary Clinton used alternate nostril breathing during her 2016 presidential campaign. Traditional yogic texts state that the alternating (switching between nostrils) nature of the breath will balance both hemispheres of the brain, while the slow nature of the breath will relax your nervous system and shift brainwaves from higher, more active states (beta waves) to relaxed flow states (alpha waves).

- Start in a seated position, sitting up straight.
- First, begin by performing 40–60 seconds of Energizer Bunny (page 109) or Breath of Fire (page 107).
- Rest your left hand palm down on your left knee, moving your right hand toward your nose.
- Place your index and middle fingers on the space between your eyebrows.
- Place your right thumb on your right nostril and your ring and pinkie fingers on the left nostril.
- Close your eyes.
- Using your right thumb, close your right nostril.
- Breathe out through your left nostril for a count of 4–5 seconds (BV 3).
- Keep holding your right nostril closed and breathe in through your left nostril for 4–5 seconds (BV 8), then close it using your ring and pinkie fingers.
- Release the right thumb to open the right nostril.
- Breathe out through the right nostril for a count of 4–5 seconds (BV 3).
- With the right nostril still open, breathe in for 4–5 seconds (BV 8), then close it using your thumb.
- Release your ring and pinkie finger to open the left nostril and breathe out for a count of 4–5 seconds (BV 3).
- Repeat 5–10 of these cycles—a full cycle is in and out of both nostrils.

Focus and concentration

In a world where our attention is being pulled in every direction all the time, you may be out of practice and find it difficult to give your full attention to just one thing. But when you are able to focus properly, you will experience a feeling of being "in the zone." In this state you make connections quickly and solutions to problems just seem to come to you. You aren't feeling stressed, but you also aren't feeling too relaxed, you are "locked in."

If you were to measure your brainwave activity in this state, you would most likely see dominance of low to mid beta brainwaves throughout parts of the brain. You aren't stressed (represented by high beta brainwaves) or daydreaming (represented by alpha brainwaves). In fact, a study conducted by Dr. Siegfried and Dr. Susan Othmer showed that using methods to reinforce beta waves (in the 15–18 Hz range) produced on average a 23 point increase in the IQ test results of participants who had been diagnosed with ADHD.[12]

This technique aims to create that same balance between feeling energized and relaxed. We will combine your favorite energizing technique (either Energizer Bunny [page 109] or Breath of Fire [page 107]) to create some energy and alertness, followed by coherent breathing (page 112) to ground the energy and balance the nervous system.

- Start in a seated position.
- First, begin by performing 40–60 seconds of Energizer Bunny (page 109) or Breath of Fire (page 107).
- Then just relax the breath and take a few seconds to notice any feelings or sensations in your body.
- Then use coherent breathing (page 112) for 3 minutes, or longer if you prefer.

Meditation

When creating Breathwork routines, one of my discoveries is that performing a stimulating and activating breathing technique before doing a relaxing and calming one actually amplifies the effectiveness of the calming technique. We can take advantage of this phenomenon to begin a meditation practice.

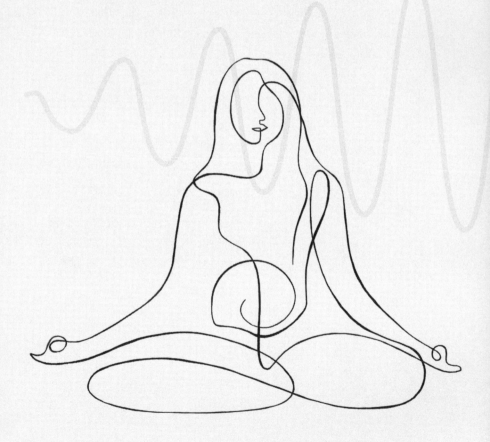

This routine is to be done before you meditate. It will quickly shift you into a deeply calm state and act as a speed ramp into your meditation practice, so you don't need to spend the first 5–10 minutes trying to get into your meditative state.

- Start in a seated position.
- Inhale through your mouth (BV 8) for 2 seconds (do not purse your lips; let your mouth relax and hang open—there should be at least 1 finger width of space between your teeth).
- Exhale through your mouth (BV 5) for 1 second, without force or control (it should feel like you are dumping the exhale out of you—you aren't trying to make it happen, it happens for you).
- Repeat this pattern for 2 minutes.

NOTE: If you start to feel dizzy, light-headed, or get some tingling in your hands/feet/face, this is a completely normal reaction as your physiology starts to change. If it becomes too uncomfortable, stop the exercise. However, if you can learn to relax into it and even enjoy the sensations, the benefits will be there for you.

- Now switch to breathing through your nose—use either breath awareness (page 102) or coherent breathing (page 112) for 3 minutes.

- Resume your normal meditation practice. If you don't have a meditation practice, continue to use breath awareness, as it is a foundational technique of many meditation methods.

SPORTS PERFORMANCE

Experience the benefits of nasal breathing

Earlier in this book we talked about the general health benefits of nasal breathing, but did you know that maintaining nasal breathing while exercising could also improve your athletic performance?

Think about the last time you exercised, whether it was running, cycling, rowing, Crossfit, boxing, or playing tennis. Were you breathing through your nose or your mouth?

As our metabolic demands become higher, it's completely natural for us to ventilate faster, usually through our mouth. There's nothing wrong with breathing through the mouth for short periods of time when the metabolic demands require it. However, new training protocols are now being developed to help develop aerobic capacity by withholding breathing through the mouth for as long as is comfortable and continuing to nasal breathe.

The know on NO

Once thought to be a toxic gas, nitric oxide (NO) was declared "Molecule of the year" by the respected journal *Science* in 1992. Our bodies naturally produce nitric oxide, primarily in the inner layer of blood vessels and our nasal cavity. It acts as an important signaling molecule, transmitting signals to cells in the cardiovascular, nervous, and immune systems.

Much research has been conducted on its role in the human body and more recently in its involvement in optimizing athletic involvement. Many athletic supplements contain ingredients that are said to increase nitric oxide production, such as nitrate or the amino acids L-citrulline and L-arginine. When breathing through the nose, nitric oxide is released in the nasal airways and transported through the lower airways and lungs.

From a cardiovascular perspective, nitric oxide is a vasodilator, meaning it supports the expansion of the blood vessels and increases the delivery of blood and oxygen to working muscles during exercise, therefore enhancing exercise performance. It will help to open up airways by dilating the smooth muscle layer of the airways, allowing for more effective transfer of oxygen to and from the lungs during exercise.

Try this

Next time you're going for a run or walking, see if you can breathe only through your nose. If you start to feel you're short of breath, rather than switching to breathing through your mouth, slow down the pace or intensity of your exercise and breathe more deeply through your nose until you catch your breath. You may find that you'll have to reduce your athletic intensity or output to match your breathing. This may be a little frustrating at first, but after a couple of weeks of this training your body will adapt and you'll start to reap the benefits of nasal breathing.

Simulating high-altitude training in your own back yard

In 2019, the Nobel prize in physiology or medicine went to three scientists for their research into how the body responds to changes in oxygen levels and how cells can sense falling oxygen levels and respond by making new blood cells.

When oxygen is in short supply, a protein complex called hypoxia-inducible factor (HIF) builds up in nearly all the cells in the body. This increase in HIF in the cells produces a number of effects, including increasing the activity of a gene used to produce erythropoietin (EPO), a hormone that boosts the creation of oxygen-carrying red blood cells.

Athletes have been using methods of training at high altitudes as a way to condition their body to low levels of oxygen and increase their count of red blood cells. This is so that, when they compete at lower altitudes, they will still have a higher concentration of red blood cells, giving them a competitive advantage. But not everybody has access to a mountain or hyperbaric chamber (a chamber that can control air pressure and simulate different altitudes).

So, is there really a way to simulate this training right in your own environment? Patrick McKeown's

Oxygen Advantage® technique has helped athletes improve their sports performance, daily well-being, and health.

Widely regarded as one of the world's leading breathing re-education experts, Patrick has trained thousands of people around the world in his technique. It teaches a new way to breathe, combined with specific exercises, such as breath-holding training—also known as hypoxia training—to optimize blood chemistry and athletic performance.

Practicing breath-holding while walking is one of the basic hypoxia training exercises that Patrick teaches to his students. While this can be slowly built up to jogging or running, it must be done slowly and preferably with guidance from a qualified expert.

Safety notice:

Long breath-holding exercises should not be performed if you are pregnant or suffer from any of the following conditions:

- Epilepsy
- Uncontrolled blood pressure levels
- Sickle cell anemia
- Any severe heart problems in the past 6 months

If you are unsure whether this is safe for you, please consult your doctor.

- This exercise will require you to hold your breath as you walk.
- If you're just beginning with this exercise, it's very important that you approach it in a cautious manner and don't over-do it. Listen to your body!
- Start to walk at a normal pace.
- After 1 minute, gently exhale and pinch your nose to hold your breath.
- If you feel uncomfortable pinching your nose while walking in public, you can simply hold your breath without holding your nose.

- Continue to walk while holding your breath, counting the paces, until you feel a medium to strong air shortage.
- Release your nose and inhale through it while continuing to walk.
- Minimize your breathing by taking very short breaths for 15 seconds. Then allow your breathing to return to normal.
- Continue walking for 30 seconds.
- Repeat this cycle of breath-holding and walking 8 to 10 times.
- NOTE: In order for your body to adapt to lower levels of oxygen, it's important to hold your breath until you feel a medium hunger for air for the first 2–3 breath holds. After that, you can challenge yourself for the remaining breath holds.
- At first, you may only be able to hold your breath for 20–30 paces before you feel a strong air shortage—even less if you have asthma or are out of breath. With repetition over time, you'll find yourself being able to hold your breath for 80 to 100 paces. Ideally your breathing will return to being calm and easy within 3 or 4 breaths. While this exercise is a challenge, it should not be stressful.

For more exercises like this and to learn more about Patrick and the Oxygen Advantage®, head to https://oxygenadvantage.com.

Post-workout recovery

You've finished work after a long day and you want to work out. So you hit the gym around 7:30 p.m. You're done with your workout by 8:30 and then head home. You have dinner, watch a bit of TV, while scrolling through your social media feeds, then decide it's time to hit the hay around 11. Your head hits the pillow and, even though your body feels tired, for the next little while you just can't stop tossing and turning. You feel completely awake and restless.

Your nervous system is still in action mode after the workout and hasn't yet switched into its relaxation mode. Luckily, we can use our breathing to shift our state rapidly into relaxation. If you do this breathing technique right after your workout, your body can go into its restoration process right away and help with physical recovery.

So, after your next workout, dedicate just a few minutes to lie or sit down, close your eyes, and breathe. Whether it's in the stretching area of the gym, or in your stationary car, or on a bus trip back home, your body and mind will thank you for it. Simply pick your favorite relaxation technique in Chapter 4 and repeat the breath for 8–10 minutes.

PHYSICAL HEALTH

Better sex

In case you didn't know already, sex is not an intellectual pursuit. Being completely present with your partner is key to fully experiencing and enjoying these intimate experiences. The quickest way to becoming more present during sex is to use your breath. There's a reason why breath is central to many of the sexual practices detailed in ancient arts, such as Tantra and Taoism.

You can use your breath to bring all your awareness into your body, generate and move sexual energy. and also turn down the volume of thoughts that might be judging, questioning, criticizing, or worrying. When you get good at doing this, your bodily feelings and sensations will begin to heighten and become more intense, as you open yourself up to all the rich and exquisite experiences that sex has to offer.

This breath can be performed while intimate with a partner. However, practice it by yourself first, while masturbating, so you get the hang of it and it starts to feel natural and easy. The last thing you want is to have to focus too much on your breathing while you're making love.

This breath is split into two parts.

Part 1—Stoking the fire

- Start in a lying position.
- Inhale slowly through your nose or mouth (usually between 4 and 6 seconds) and visualize your breath traveling all the way down to your genitals.
- As you exhale through your mouth, keep your attention on your genitals, noticing any sensation or even a thought or emotion that appears in this area.
- The exhale is a release. No effort to push air out, just relax your body.
- Keep your breath moving. Do not pause between inhales or exhales.
- Repeat this breath 10 times.

Part 2—The pleasure wheel

- Inhale slowly through your nose or mouth (usually between 4 and 6 seconds) and visualize that you are drawing energy from your genitals up the back of your spine all the way to the crown of your head. Imagine the energy moving through your body as pleasure, arousal, or just good feelings.
- As you exhale through your mouth, visualize that energy moving back down the front of your spine to your genitals.

- With every inhale and exhale, you're creating an elongated loop or wheel starting at your genitals, extending to the crown of your head, and then looping back to your genitals.
- Keep your breath moving. Do not pause between inhales or exhales.
- Keep paying attention to the feelings and sensations in your body. How much can you feel the sensations? Can you notice any emotions or thoughts?
- Continue for 5–10 minutes, or just keep going, because it can feel so good!

You can even try this technique with a partner BEFORE you are intimate, although don't be surprised if you just want to jump on each other before you finish the technique!

Breathe together!

A beautiful way to connect deeply with your partner is to breathe together. Next time you are in bed, try spooning with your partner and feel their breathing against your body. Try to synchronize to the rhythm of their breathing, noticing the differences in speed and length. You can also do this facing each other while gazing into each other's eyes, which provides another layer to a very deep experience.

Anne already enjoyed a very pleasurable sex life with her husband. She came to a guided Breathwork class that I was teaching in a meditation studio in London, simply interested in trying something new and learning how to find calm in her busy life. During the experience, the breath led her awareness into her body, causing her to notice sensations like she had never had before—she had never felt so connected to her body. The next time she was intimate with her husband, she was so much more in tune with her body and instantly started to notice new feelings and sensations that she had never previously felt—like electricity running through her entire body, resulting in the most mind-blowing orgasm she had ever experienced.

Quitting smoking

For many smokers, having a cigarette or a smoke break is the only time they give themselves to do nothing but breathe consciously. They will take about 5 minutes to take long and slow breaths, so maybe it's not just the cigarette making them feel relaxed, it's the way they are breathing!

Once you've decided to quit, use this exercise whenever you feel the urge to smoke and you'll see that you don't need the cigarette!

- Start standing or seated.
- Inhale through pursed lips the same way that you would through a cigarette—you can even bring your fingers to your lips.
- Usually, this inhale will last between 3 and 4 seconds. As you inhale, really focus on breathing diaphragmatically and sense the air being pulled all the way down into the bottom of your lungs.
- Exhale through your mouth in the same way that you would when you smoke and maybe even a little longer (maybe between 4 and 5 seconds).
- Pause for 1–2 seconds.
- Continue this for 5 minutes.

- If you like, you could even go through a ritual of imagining opening a cigarette pack, taking one out, lighting it, and holding it in your fingers. Over time you won't need to do this any more. But if it helps you in the beginning, go for it.

A note on other addictions:

For addictions to other substances, such as alcohol or other drugs, I would always suggest that people try the integrative styles of Breathwork (page 193) alongside professional help where necessary.

Headaches and migraines

This technique is called Butterfly Breathing and can be used in the middle of a headache or migraine, to great effect.

It will involve you softly breathing in and out through your nose in a connected way. Once you reach the top of your inhale, you'll turn straight into your exhale without pause. Once you reach the bottom of your exhale, turn straight into your inhale without pause. The breaths will be small and your exhale is relaxed.

- Inhale through your nose (BV 6–7).
- Without pause, exhale through your nose (BV 5).
- Continue this breath without any pauses between the inhales and exhales.
- As you breathe, start to scan your body for any physical tension (e.g., in the muscles or joints). On the inhale, focus on breathing into these areas, and on the exhale, focus on relaxing and releasing these areas.
- Once you have gone through your entire body, now think of a moment in your life, a person, or a thing that makes you feel love, joy, warmth, or gratitude, or just really, really good. Keep the rate of your breathing consistent.

- When you think of this feeling, give it a color—
  whichever one pops into your head first.
- On your next inhale, send the breath into the
  epicenter of the pain in your head and fill this space
  with the color that you have picked.
- As you exhale, just relax and release any tension that
  you may feel (you can even visualize releasing tension
  in your brain).
- Repeat this breath, filling your head with this
  pleasurable color on the inhale; then relaxing and
  letting go of any pain or tension on the exhale—for
  10 minutes or however long you need.

NOTE: At some point you may feel like you want to
take a deeper breath. If this happens, let it happen!
Give yourself a couple of sighs of relief (page 129), then
go straight back into the Butterfly Breaths.

Asthma

If you suffer from asthma and are interested in a drug-free approach to healing, the Buteyko method is a great place to start. Konstantin Buteyko was a Ukrainian-born Russian physiologist who stated that many health problems (including asthma) come as a result of people breathing too much, leading to chronic hypocapnia, as discussed on page 46. According to Buteyko, asthma is not a disease but it is the body trying to preserve carbon dioxide levels in the blood. So the Buteyko method is designed to reduce over-breathing, using a series of exercises.

The breath-holding exercises that you do in your Core 15 and Focus 5 programs either come from the Buteyko method or are Buteyko inspired. If you are looking to work on your asthma, choose the Focus 5 program for CO_2 tolerance and practice this daily.

If you would like to find out more about the Buteyko method, I would highly recommend the work of Patrick McKeown, one of the world's leading Buteyko practitioners: https://buteykoclinic.com.

Asthma can be an emotional business

Alongside the physiological approaches to treating asthma, it's also important to acknowledge the potential emotional link between breathing difficulties, including the role of skeletal muscle tension, especially in the primary breathing muscles such as the diaphragm as a result of stress, anxiety, and emotional trauma. Integrative styles of Breathwork can be used in therapeutic ways to release these tensions and reduce asthma symptoms.

Refer to page 193 to learn more about the Breathwork styles that can be useful in these instances.

High blood pressure (hypertension)

Search online and you'll find page after page of breathing techniques that can help reduce hypertension. What all these techniques will have in common is a slowing down of the breath. Research conducted in 2005 by the American Heart Association found that mindfully breathing more slowly can reduce sympathetic activity (the stress response), heart rate, and blood pressure.[13]

- Choose your favorite de-stress technique (starting at page 110).
- Perform it at least 3 times a day (e.g., morning, before lunch, before bed) for at least 5 minutes.

Pain

Research conducted by the University of Regensburg has shown how relaxed and slow breathing when in pain can help you process the negative emotions that go along with it.[14]

Visualization has also been found to improve pain processing—the mind has an amazing ability to create a more relaxed state and release natural happy hormones (endorphins), helping to reduce the negative impact of pain. When you put the two together, you have a fantastic tool to manage your own pain.

An important note while you do this exercise is not to try to focus on making the pain go away. Just focus on relaxing and create comfort in that moment. The results may just surprise you!

- Start in a seated or lying position.
- First, pick a color that represents soothing, healing and relaxation for you.
- Inhale through your nose for 4 seconds (BV 8). As you inhale, visualize that you are drawing this color through your nose, down through your throat into your lungs and then sending it to wherever you have

pain, surrounding and engulfing the pain point
completely.

- The pain point may have a color, in which case
  completely encase this color with your soothing
  color.
- Exhale through the mouth for 8 seconds (BV 3). As
  you exhale, visualize that the soothing color is
  grabbing the pain and pulling it out of you as you
  exhale it out.
- Repeat this pattern for at least 10 minutes, or as long
  as you need until the pain is at a bearable level or
  gone completely!

NOTE: If you have a chronic pain condition, there are
other Breathwork techniques you can use, such as the
Wim Hof Method (page 178) or the integrative styles of
Breathwork (page 193).

Hangovers

Alcohol dials up your sympathetic nervous system. The effect of excess alcohol in your body means you'll become dehydrated and inflamed, with less blood sugar and excess stomach acids and toxic substances.

Next time you're feeling a bit dusty, blow away the booze with this breathing technique. It will promote movement of lymph through your body and stimulate your digestive system to dramatically increase the elimination of waste products. It will also lightly increase adrenaline, which causes more glucose to be available in your bloodstream.

- Start in a seated or lying position.
- Inhale through your mouth (BV 8) for 2 seconds.
- Do not purse your lips, let your mouth relax and hang open—there should be at least 1 finger width of space between your teeth.
- Remember your diaphragmatic breathing—this is important for stimulating your digestive organs.
- Exhale through your mouth (BV 5) for 1 second without force or control. It should feel like you are dumping the exhale out of you. You aren't trying to make it happen, it happens for you.
- Repeat this pattern for 2 minutes.

NOTE: If you start to feel dizzy, light-headed, or get some tingling in your hands/feet/face, this is a completely normal reaction as your physiology starts to change. If it becomes too uncomfortable, stop the exercise. However, if you can learn to relax into it and even enjoy the sensations, the benefits will be there for you.

- After the final breath, take a deep breath in through your mouth (BV 9), then hold your breath and slowly count backward from 15.
- Once you get to 0, exhale (BV 5), then hold your breath again and slowly count backward from 15.
- Relax and take a few slow breaths.
- When you feel ready, repeat this pattern of breathing and breath-holding again.
- If you feel like you want to, you can do it a third time as well!

Nausea and motion sickness

A 2014 study conducted by the University of Kentucky put participants through a virtual reality (VR) motion sickness experience to test whether conscious breathing could reduce symptoms. The group that was taught how to use conscious breathing throughout the experience showed a significant increase in parasympathetic tone and reported fewer motion sickness symptoms than the control group.[15]

Couple this with a grounding visualization and you have a sure-fire way to relieve your queasiness. This technique has worked so well with people suffering motion sickness, people going through chemotherapy, and pregnant women.

- Start in a standing or seated position.
- Inhale through the nose for 4 seconds (BV 8), focusing on breathing diaphragmatically.
- As you inhale, visualize the breath traveling from your nose all the way down to the soles of your feet.
- Envisage roots growing out of the soles of your feet, running deep into the earth. With every inhale, watch the roots get bigger and stronger and travel deeper into the earth.
- Exhale through the mouth with pursed lips for a count of 8 (BV 3).
- Continue until the queasiness has passed.

THE WIM HOF METHOD (WHM)

From climbing Everest and Kilimanjaro in nothing but shorts and shoes to running the fastest barefoot half marathon on ice and snow, to running a full marathon in the Namib Desert without water, Wim Hof has captured the world's attention and fascination just by how he does it! And, of course, breathing is a big part of it.

As you've read at the beginning of the book, the WHM is where my Breathwork journey began. Over the years, I have seen person after person gain profound benefits from a consistent practice of this method.

Since there are so many different potential physical, mental, and emotional benefits from this practice, I'm going to tell a few stories of people who I've either met or worked with who have experienced great success with the WHM.

Autoimmune (AI) diseases

The immune system is one of your body's lines of defense to guard you against foreign invaders like bacteria and viruses. Normally, the immune system is effective in telling the difference between foreign cells and your own cells. When you have an AI disease, your immune system mistakes part of your body, such as your joints or skin, as foreign and starts to attack your body.

My journey to finding Breathwork started when my dad was diagnosed with MS, an AI disease that damages the protective coating that surrounds nerve cells, called the myelin sheath. Since then, I've witnessed many other people have great success with the WHM in all types of AI diseases. But how can the WHM be useful in the treatment of AI diseases? We can't influence our immune system consciously. Or, can we?

Wim claimed his techniques allowed him to have influence over his immune system and was willing to put them to the test in a laboratory setting. In a controlled experiment, researchers injected him with an endotoxin (a dead bacteria) that would normally cause a human's immune system to react in flu-like symptoms, including fever, shivering, and headaches. But when they injected Wim while he was doing his breathing techniques, he experienced no symptoms at all.

Researchers decided to repeat the experiment with 24 young and healthy male volunteers. Twelve of the volunteers spent a week learning the WHM, while the other 12 did not. All the volunteers were injected with the same endotoxin. The group that had no training experienced a range of reactions from mild symptoms to strong fever, while the group who had learned the WHM experienced no symptoms.

Blood work from the group that had learned the WHM showed that, immediately after they started applying the method, they had increased levels of adrenaline. Also, the anti-inflammatory protein IL-10 repressed levels of the inflammatory proteins IL-6, IL-8 and TNF-Alpha. The results from this experiment suggest that we have the ability to consciously down-regulate our inflammatory response, something that could prove to be very useful in the treatment of autoimmune diseases.

Diet and mindset

If you want to tackle an autoimmune disease head on, I would suggest that looking at your nutrition and mindset is critical to your recovery. My dad followed the Wahls protocol diet for many years, which helped him immensely (https://terrywahls.com/diet). I also believe that maintaining a positive mindset is critical to recovery. One of my favorite books that I recommend to everyone is *Breaking the Habit of Being Yourself*, by Dr. Joe Dispenza. It combines the fields of quantum physics, neuroscience, brain chemistry, biology, and genetics to give the necessary knowledge and tools to make measurable changes in your life.

Endometriosis

Endometriosis is a condition that affects an estimated 1 in 10 women during their reproductive years. It occurs when tissue similar to the inner lining of the uterus (endometrium) grows outside the uterus, where it can cause chronic inflammation and build-up of scar tissue. This results in symptoms such as painful menstruation, heavy bleeding, chronic pelvic pain, and infertility. While there's no known cure for endometriosis, it can be treated through various medications and surgical interventions. However, success rates vary significantly.

While research still needs to be conducted, there is anecdotal evidence where daily practice of the WHM has been useful in reducing and even reversing symptoms—most likely because of its effect on the endocrine system (the collection of glands that produce and regulate hormones) and its ability to reduce inflammatory cytokines (signaling molecules that promote inflammation).

Jennifer suffered from severe endometriosis that had overtaken one of her ovaries and was blocking the second. She experienced constant pain and bloating and the chance of her having children was unlikely. She underwent five laparoscopic surgeries to remove the excess endometrium from the outside of her uterus, but it kept growing back. In her fifth and last surgery, the gynecologist ended the surgery soon after it commenced, later stating that there was no point doing any more work as she was never going to be able to have children naturally. This was obviously devastating news, but she didn't give up. Her husband had already been doing the WHM daily and he suggested that Jennifer give it a go. Jennifer began a daily regime of breathing exercises and cold showers. Twelve weeks after starting the method, she fell pregnant naturally. The couple now have two children and Jennifer is completely symptom free.

Chronic pain and fatigue

Chronic pain and fatigue conditions are mysterious, misunderstood, and can be soul crushing for anyone who experiences them. The three most common pain and fatigue conditions are myalgic encephalomyelitis (ME), chronic fatigue syndrome (CFS), and fibromyalgia (FM). It is estimated that as many as 17–24 million people worldwide experience ME/CFS.

Research to understand the causes of these conditions continues. Current theories range from viral infection, central nervous system dysfunction, genetics, immune dysfunction, emotional stress, and trauma, and a range of treatments and therapies exists to help those suffering. From my experience working with clients suffering from these conditions, I have found that a daily practice of the WHM can be transformative and really help reduce symptoms and aid recovery.

While there are several reasons this helps, I believe the main reason is that, by consciously manipulating your breathing, you are affecting your autonomic nervous system. The constant stress and frustration of these conditions takes its toll emotionally and at a nervous system level, creating a constant and overactive "fight or flight" response. Doing the

WHM teaches the nervous system how to go back into its parasympathetic operation, promoting recovery and restoration.

Carly suffered from ME for 3 years. She was constantly exhausted through joint pain and would spend all her free time resting in bed. Daily headaches and feeling unwell disrupted her school and work life. Leaving the house was always planned days in advance, so that she could "prepare." She would have to rest in bed a day before and 2 days after. If she pushed herself too much, she would undo months of progress toward her recovery.

Since practicing the WHM method, Carly is no longer in pain nor in a constant state of fatigue. While she may still experience fatigue when she overexerts herself, it is immediately improved by WHM breathing. She no longer feels constantly unwell or has headaches, and can now work full-time and leave the house spontaneously. Although she looks forward to her breathing sessions and daily cold showers, the biggest change is in her mindset. Carly is now a lot more positive about her future and believes that she will make a full recovery.

Irritable bowel syndrome (IBS)

IBS is quite a common condition that affects the gut and causes symptoms such as bloating, stomach cramps, constipation, and diarrhea. IBS can be very frustrating to live with and there's currently no cure, but you can manage symptoms through changes in diet and various medicines.

My experience working with clients is that IBS and stress and anxiety go hand in hand. It's not totally clear how they are related, or which comes first, but studies show they likely happen together.[16] This may be because being constantly in "fight or flight" mode decreases digestive and/or immune function. The WHM can help those with IBS by decreasing inflammation and inducing feelings of ease, peace, and calm. The diaphragmatic nature of the breath also helps to massage and stimulate the digestive organs.

Slow breathing

We know that our digestive system is functioning best when we are in our parasympathetic or "rest and digest" state. So go back to Chapter 4 and pick your favorite stress release technique—do this for 3–5 minutes before you eat a meal to relax your nervous system and prime your belly for food.

Altitude sickness

At higher altitudes, each breath you take contains fewer oxygen molecules. At roughly 18,000 feet, each breath contains about half of the amount of oxygen that would be found at sea level. In order to compensate for this, you will naturally breathe faster and your heart has to work harder. But generally, your blood oxygen levels will still not be up to the same concentration as at sea level.

On average, the human body needs between 1 and 3 days to acclimatize to higher altitudes. This gives your body enough time to respond to the change in altitude by altering lung pressure, blood pH levels, and electrolyte, salt, and fluid levels. If you don't give your body time to acclimatize, you may experience symptoms of altitude sickness (also known as acute mountain sickness) such as dizziness, exhaustion, insomnia, shortness of breath, and nausea or vomiting. If ignored, extreme cases can even lead to death.

While at altitude, taking moments to sit/lie down and do rounds of the WHM can help significantly. The focused deep breathing will help to top up blood oxygen levels, and breath-holding will promote the production of more oxygen-carrying red blood cells. This is what allowed Wim Hof to lead an expedition of 18 amateur trekkers up to the summit of Mount Kilimanjaro (19,341 feet above sea level), setting a Guinness World Record group time of 31 hours and 25 minutes, with no reported signs of altitude sickness.

HOW TO DO
THE WHM BREATHING TECHNIQUE

I usually recommend doing this technique in the morning before eating any food.

For the WHM, there are a few important safety points that must be observed.

- Only perform these exercises in a safe environment. Don't do the breathing exercises in or around water or while driving any vehicle.
- The effects of these exercises can be intense. Please go at your own pace; no need to push yourself too fast.
- These exercises should not be done by pregnant women or persons with epilepsy, uncontrolled blood pressure levels, sickle cell anemia, or who have had any severe heart problems in the past 6 months.
- If you have a health condition and you are unsure if this is safe for you, please consult a physician.

- Start in a seated or lying position.
- Inhale deeply through your nose or mouth.
- Exhale through your mouth without force or control.
- It should feel like the exhale is just falling out of you. Don't try to speed it up or slow it down.
- This is 1 breath cycle. Repeat for 30 breath cycles.

NOTE: If you start to feel dizzy, light-headed, or get some tingling in your hands/feet/face, this is a completely normal reaction, as your physiology starts to change. If it becomes too uncomfortable, stop the exercise. However, if you can learn to relax into it and enjoy the sensations, the benefits will be there for you.

- On your final breath, exhale and then hold your breath (don't breathe in and hold).
- When you feel a strong urge to breathe, take a deep breath in and then hold that breath in (lungs full) for 10 to 15 seconds.
- Then relax and exhale.
- Take a moment or two to sense what you feel in your body.
- This is one round. Repeat this round twice more, to make a total of 3 rounds.

- Once you have completed 3 rounds, just take a moment to relax and enjoy the state that you have created for yourself.

HOW TO DO THE COLD EXPOSURE

Wim encourages you to gradually expose yourself to the cold—no need to force anything too quickly.

- Start just by simply taking cold showers every morning. Even just 30 seconds is a fantastic start—switch the shower to cold for the final moments.
- The important thing, when you're in the cold shower, is not to tense up. Relax your muscles, slow down your breathing, and become like a jellyfish drifting in the ocean.
- To learn more about Wim Hof and his techniques, visit www.wimhofmethod .com.

INTEGRATIVE BREATHWORK

THE EXTRAORDINARY HEALING POWER OF THE BREATH

Always driven to find out what other benefits were possible with Breathwork, my continuous exploration eventually brought me to the various methods that are categorized as Integrative Breathwork—in my opinion, one of the most exciting potentials of Breathwork.

As I continued to learn from great teachers, experts, and masters, I became convinced that as more people learn about these methods and understand what they can do for them, our world will change in a big way.

Integrative Breathwork is a category of Breathwork focused on emotional healing and spiritual exploration and development. My experiences in Integrative Breathwork have enabled me to completely let go of past experiences and traumas that had continued to haunt me, even if I hadn't realized it! It has given me a greater understanding of who I am and the nature of the universe, and has even provided glimpses into the mystical realms of consciousness and the supernatural.

Integrative Breathwork uses methods of breathing to safely shift your awareness and your body's physiology to induce what Dr. Stan Groff, creator of Holotropic Breathwork, calls "non-ordinary states of consciousness." It is in these states that powerful and transformative physical, mental, emotional, and spiritual healing can occur.

Non-ordinary states have been used by ancient and aboriginal cultures since time immemorial—as a rite of passage, for healing and spiritual exploration—using methods such as chanting, dancing, breathing, meditation, heat exposure, fasting, and psychedelic plants. For the longest time, mainstream scientists dismissed the value of these practices. However, now there is much research by institutions such as the Multidisciplinary Association for Psychedelic Studies (MAPS) and the Centre for Psychedelic Research at Imperial College London, aimed at understanding and uncovering the potential healing benefits of non-ordinary states, particularly for conditions such as PTSD, depression, ADHD, and chronic anxiety.

Through Integrative Breathwork, I have witnessed so many people have massive breakthroughs in their own healing, including overcoming grief, liberation from past traumas, feeling confident to come off anti-anxiety medication, and finding permanent relief from physical pain.

Below are just a few of my more extraordinary personal experiences during my own Breathwork journey.

Transformational Breath in Antalya, Turkey

I attended a weeklong training with Judith Kravitz, the creator of a Breathwork method called Transformational Breath. Judith first experienced conscious Breathwork in the mid-seventies, through the breathing practice known as Rebirthing. She then integrated various other healing tools, including movement, toning, and body mapping, to create Transformational Breath.

In this training, Judith explained how using a "full circular breathing pattern" activates a high frequency through the body's energy systems. Through the principle of entrainment, any remaining low frequency energy patterns resulting from past traumas are raised in the presence of the higher frequency energy state, to clear blockages within the energy system. To be honest, at that moment I really didn't understand what that meant but I was open to the experience.

During one of the sessions, as I lay on the floor breathing in this circular pattern, my mind was transported back to a time when I was about 9 years old. I was a bit of a mischievous child and on the rare occasion where I would push the line and do something particularly naughty, my father would give me a little slap on the bottom as a punishment. In one such moment, I'd done something particularly reckless and in the heat of the moment, my father struck me harder than he ever had before, rocking me into a state of shock.

As soon as this memory entered my awareness, what followed were massive waves of emotion—sadness, confusion, injustice, and betrayal. I had no idea that that small event in my life held some emotional charge over me and may have been unconsciously affecting me in some way. But, here I was, crying, screaming, with my whole body uncontrollably flailing about of its own accord. After maybe a minute or so, the emotion passed and this deep sense of lightness, calm, and peace came over me, remaining with me for the rest of the week. I felt somehow different, like the world seemed a little bit brighter and lighter.

Rebirthing in Baja California, Mexico

Created by Leonard Orr and commonly agreed as one of the two original Western therapeutic methods of Breathwork developed out of the 1970s, Rebirthing is the home of "conscious connected breathing," a technique of breathing that many schools of Integrative Breathwork now adopt.

I have had the good fortune to be trained in Rebirthing by one of Leonard's first students, now a legend in the Breathwork world, Dan Brulé. I stayed with Dan for one month in an off-the-grid community, Baja Biosana, in Baja California, Mexico. Each day we breathed and each session brought a new breakthrough or insight for me. In one particular session, the face of an Indian saint came into my awareness. As I stared at his kind face, gently grinning at me, I felt incredible waves of love, care, and acceptance flow through my body and I started to cry out of sheer love and joy. My sense was that he was giving me a blessing or encouragement. A message like, "You are perfect as you are, you can do it!" just kept washing over me, overwhelming me completely.

After what felt like hours, I heard Dan's voice in the background saying to start slowing down my breath and relax. Although I didn't want this moment to end, it was time to return to normal consciousness. The face smiled at me and, before I could think another thought, it zoomed forward toward me and merged into my body. Instantly, my whole body started to vibrate uncontrollably and I started to laugh ecstatically and I could not stop for at least 15 minutes. After the breath session, I was left with a feeling of ecstatic energy, happiness, and excitement, with so much love for the blessing that is my life.

Holotropic Breathwork in Basel, Switzerland

I attended a workshop with Stanislav Grof, the creator of a Breathwork method called Holotropic Breathwork. Also considered one of the original Western therapeutic methods of Breathwork from the 1970s, Holotropic means "moving toward wholeness" (from the Greek "holos," meaning whole, and "trepein," meaning moving in the direction of something).

Deeply interested in altered states of consciousness as a potential therapeutic tool, psychiatrists Stanislav and Christina Grof developed Holotropic Breathwork, which integrates insights from modern consciousness research, anthropology, transpersonal psychology, Eastern spiritual practices, and mystical traditions of the world.

In the workshop I attended, over 150 people from all over the world were packed into one big hall (I did wonder whether there was going to be enough oxygen for us all in there!). As the Breathwork session began, people instantly started to go into their various experiences. Some people were laughing, others were crying. People were whooping with joy, or remaining quite silent and still.

Holotropic Breathwork sessions tend to be quite long, usually between 2 and 3 hours. About what felt like halfway through the session, my body started to feel very tired and I felt a lot of resistance to continuing. Rather than just deciding to stop, I opted to completely let go of whatever was happening and simply allow my breath to carry on by itself, at whatever rate and volume that it wanted. As soon as I made this decision, a feeling of lightness started around my neck and shoulders, then spread across my entire body. It felt as though I was floating up off the ground into the air, until eventually I realized that I actually was floating! Even though my eyes were closed, I was having visions of the room I was in, just as clear as though my eyes were open. I could see the room and I could see my body lying on the floor! I was able to move around the room, observing the other people breathing. This was the first of many out-of-body experiences that I have experienced during Integrative Breathwork sessions.

Biodynamic Breathwork and Trauma Release System (BBTRS) in Bali

I attended a BBTRS training with its founder, Giten Tonkov. BBTRS uses six elements which, when applied together, maximize the potential for releases of trauma and healing: breath, movement, touch, emotional expression, sound, and meditation.

Where many styles of Integrative Breathwork will begin lying down, BBTRS does things differently. To focus the direction of the session on a certain aspect of healing, a particular session might start you in a different position. What also makes BBTRS unique is its emphasis on trauma-informed body work.

During one session, where I was being facilitated (we call it getting "breathed") by a fellow trainee, Giten came to assess me. Without saying a word, he used his thumb and forefinger to gently grasp a muscle just to the side of my larynx. As he gently squeezed it, all of a sudden I felt this incredible rage start from the middle of my chest, then make its way up to my throat. There was no going back now.

Even though I screamed with anger, what came out was not my voice, but a deeper, more primal sound. While I had no idea what this rage was related to, I knew that it was something from deep within that I needed to express and release. After the Breathwork session, tension in my jaw, neck and shoulders released, my muscles felt soft like jelly and a chronic pain that I'd had in my left shoulder blade for about 6 years was 90 percent gone.

As the popularity of Breathwork continues to grow, more and more researchers are expressing interest in exploring the physiological changes that can occur using this amazing therapeutic tool. However, the anecdotal evidence is undeniable. Time and time again, I witness the remarkable, as people are able to shed layers of accumulated trauma and frozen stress and tension in their nervous system and even start to open their awareness to new levels of consciousness, often having mystical and divine experiences. When I work with clients who are experiencing Breathwork for the first time, it is not uncommon for them to place the session in the top five most significant events in their life.

There are many styles of Integrative Breathwork out there that all have their own style and use of techniques. I highly recommend you try a few to see which one agrees with you the most. Your first few sessions should be undertaken under the supervision of an experienced and qualified practitioner. I suggest searching for Breathwork practitioners near you. Here's a list of some prominent figures and schools:

- Breath Mastery with Dan Brulé—www.breathmastery.com
- Holotropic Breathwork—www.holotropic.com
- Biodynamic Breathwork and Trauma Release System—www.biodynamicbreath.com

- Transformational Breath—
  www.transformationalbreath.com
- Alchemy of Breath—www.alchemyofbreath.com
- Rebirthing Breathwork—
  www.rebirthingbreathwork.com
- Therapeutic Breathwork with Jim Morningstar—
  www.transformationsusa.com

Conclusion

What I hope you take away from this book is excitement at the possibilities and potential for yourself.

Every day I see people around the world being amazed at the power of the breath. Seeing people's expressions of disbelief at what they just experienced after a Breathwork session is one of the favorite parts of my work, because I know that I have just witnessed the beginning of a new chapter for that person.

We are continuously learning and discovering more about how brilliant the human body is and how we already possess so many of the tools that we need to improve our well-being, health, and performance.

It doesn't always take going on super restrictive diets, taking up Crossfit, meditating for 2 hours a day, or becoming a yogi for you to start to experience big changes in your life. By now you can agree that something as simple as tuning into your breath and learning how to use it in different ways can open up new dimensions of health and happiness for you.

There is such a great power in all of us wanting to be expressed, but to realize this power means reflecting on your life and deciding what needs to be done differently. The hardest part about change is not doing the same things that you did yesterday.

So can you take time out of your busy life to invest in yourself and prioritize consciously creating new small habits? You can start with practicing your Core 15 + Focus 5 (or even just parts of it if you can only spare a few minutes), or even just setting a reminder each day to check your breath (are your shoulders relaxed, are you breathing through your nose?). If you create consistency, these habits will become second nature, at which point you can focus on something new.

Your journey in life is personal to you, but it has something in common with everyone else—it's a JOURNEY! It means that making progress is as simple as focusing on taking one small step after the other and over time you will be able to look back at all the footprints you've made and smile. You will also notice many other footprints alongside yours and understand that we are all on the same journey together.

We are all individual pieces contributing to the same puzzle that is our world. If each one of us can learn to be a little more kind, loving, and compassionate, first to ourselves and then to the people around us, then, with every breath we breathe, we are all contributing to a peaceful and prosperous future on this planet.

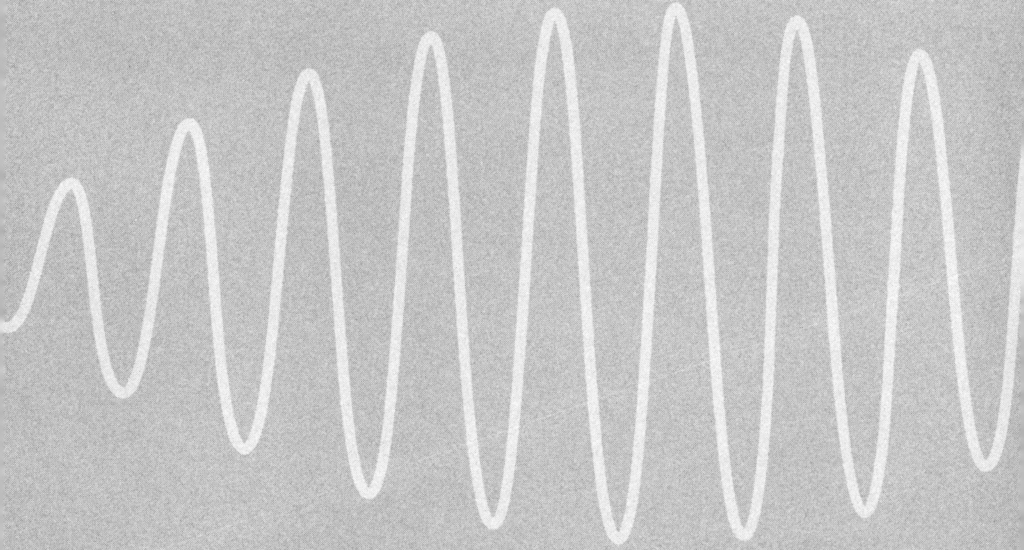

Acknowledgments

As I pen (or type) the final words in this book, it fills me with a sense of excitement, accomplishment, relief, but also sadness and grief. Over the months writing this book, it became clear to me that it represented a closing of a chapter in my life and the start of a new one. And now that the book is complete, there is a certain feeling of loss, as I say good-bye to the old and welcome the new.

Now is a time where I can reflect on what has been a magnificent, wondrous, and sometimes hard and painful journey on this earth so far and say thank you for the many blessings and gifts that have come into my life.

I have grown up in a family that is extremely close and I see this as the biggest blessing in my life. To my mom and dad, Yujin and David—I now understand why I chose you! From the bottom of my heart, thank you for your unwavering love, support, and belief in me. To my brothers, Jim and Ian— thank you for always being there for me and being such a source of brotherly support, love, and a good laugh. To Mel, Peri, Maya, Flynn, Nina, Aria, and Declan—thank you for always sharing your warmth and bringing so much love and fun into my life.

ACKNOWLEDGMENTS

I have been given so much from so many incredible teachers, both in a formal teacher–student setting and more broadly in the relationships and interactions I've had with various people who have come into my life. To all my teachers, I treasure our interaction whether it was in person, through a computer screen, through a book, or in spirit. Thank you for your wisdom, time, and energy to help me grow, whether you knew you were doing it or not!

A book only happens because of the team behind it. I want to thank the team at Penguin Life, Emily, Alice, Corinna, and Susannah, for your enthusiasm, guidance, and patience—you have been an absolute dream to work with. I also want to give a big thank-you to Jackie, who was amazing at helping me understand the world of publishing. And finally, a massive thank-you to Mark for your generous wisdom that helped me turn my whirlwind of ideas into a book I am extremely proud of.

And finally to you, the reader. Thank you for taking the time to read through the pages of this book. I hope the words contained here are of service and open up a new world of possibility for you.

References

1. Robert L. Fried, *Breathe Well, Be Well: A Program to Relieve Stress, Anxiety, Asthma, Hypertension, Migraine, and Other Disorders for Better Health*, Wiley, 1994.

2. Leon Chaitow, Dinah Bradley, and Christopher Gilbert, *Recognizing and Treating Breathing Disorders: A Multidisciplinary Approach*, Churchill Livingstone, 2nd edition, 2013.

3. Rene Cailliet and Leonard Gross, *Rejuvenation Strategy*, Doubleday & Co., 1987.

4. Mental Health Foundation, "Stressed Nation: 74% of UK 'overwhelmed or unable to cope' at some point in the past year," May 14, 2018; https://www.mentalhealth.org.uk/news /stressed-nation-74-uk-overwhelmed-or-unable-cope-some -point-past-year.

5. Stephen B. Elliott, *The New Science of Breath*, 2nd edition, Coherence Publishing, 2005.

6. R. J. S. Gerritsen and G. P. H. Band, "Breath of life: the respiratory vagal stimulation model of contemplative activity," *Frontiers in Human Neuroscience*, 2018; https://www.ncbi.nlm .nih.gov/pmc/articles/PMC6189422.

7. M. Kuppusamy et al., "Immediate effects of *Bhramari pranayama* on resting cardiovascular parameters in healthy adolescents," *Journal of Clinical and Diagnostic Research*, May 2016; https://www.ncbi.nlm.nih.gov/pmc/articles /PMC4948385.

8. E. Vlemincx et al., "Respiratory variability preceding and following sighs: a resetter hypothesis," *Biological Psychology*, 2010, 84 (1), 82–7, PMID: 19744538.

9. B. G. Kalyani et al., "Neurohemodynamic correlates of 'OM' chanting: A pilot functional magnetic resonance imaging study," *International Journal of Yoga*, 2011; https://www.ncbi.nlm.nih.gov/pmc/articles/PMC3099099.

10. C. Zelano et al., "Nasal respiration entrains human limbic oscillations and modulates cognitive function," *Journal of Neuroscience*, December 7, 2016, doi: 10.1523/JNEUROSCI.2586-16.2016.

11. C. D. B. Luft et al., "Right temporal alpha oscillations as a neural mechanism for inhibiting obvious associations," *PNAS*, December 2018; https://www.pnas.org/content/115/52/E12144.

12. S. Othmer and S. F. Othmer, "Development history of the Othmer method," http://www.eeginfo.com/research/researchpapers/Research-w-Othmer-Method-2017.pdf.

13. N. J. Chacko et al., "Slow breathing improves arterial baroreflex sensitivity and decreases blood pressure in essential hypertension," *Hypertension*, August 2005; https://www.ahajournals.org/doi/full/10.1161/01.hyp.0000179581.68566.7d.

14. V. Busch et al., "The effect of deep and slow breathing on pain perception, autonomic activity, and mood processing—a study," *Pain Medicine*, 2012; https://www.ncbi.nlm.nih.gov/pubmed/21939499.

15. M. E. Russell et al., "Use of controlled diaphragmatic breathing for the management of motion sickness in a virtual reality environment," *Applied Psychophysiology and Biofeedback*, December 2014; https://www.ncbi.nlm.nih.gov/pubmed/25280524.

16. H. Qin et al., "Impact of psychological stress on irritable bowel syndrome," *World Journal of Gastroenterology*, October 2014; https://www.ncbi.nlm.nih.gov/pmc/articles/PMC4202343.

Further reading

Corrective Breathwork

Leon Chaitow, Dinah Bradley, and Christopher Gilbert, *Recognising and Treating Breathing Disorders: A Multidisciplinary Approach*, Churchill Livingstone, 2nd edition, 2013.

Donna Farhi, *The Breathing Book: Good Health and Vitality Through Essential Breathwork*, Holt Paperbacks, 1996.

Patrick McKeown, *Close Your Mouth: Breathing Clinic Self-Help Manual*, Gardners Books, 2003.

Belisa Vranich, *Breathe: The Simple Revolutionary 14-Day Program to Improve Your Mental and Physical Health*, Griffin, 2016.

Integrative Breathwork

Stanislav Grof and Christina Grof, *Holotropic Breathwork: A New Approach to Self-Exploration and Therapy*, Excelsior Editions, 2010.

Judith Kravitz, *Beathe Deep Laugh Loudly: The Joy of Transformational Breathing*, Trafford Publishing, 2007.

Jim Morningstar, *Break Through with Breathwork: Jumpstarting Personal Growth in Counseling and the Healing Arts*, North Atlantic Books, 2017.

Leonard Orr with Sondra Ray, *Rebirthing in the New Age*, Celestial Arts, 1977.

Giten Tonkov, *Feel to Heal: Releasing Trauma Through Body Awareness and Breathwork Practice*, independently published, 2019.

Mind–body Breathwork

Richard P. Brown and Patricia L. Gerbarg, *The Healing Power of The Breath: Simple Techniques to Reduce Stress and Anxiety, Enhance Concentration, and Balance Your Emotions*, Shambhala, 2012.

Dan Brulé, *Just Breathe: Mastering Breathwork for Success in Life, Love, Business, and Beyond*, Atria/Enliven Books, 2017.

Robert L. Fried, *Breathe Well, Be Well: A Program to Relieve Stress, Anxiety, Asthma, Hypertension, Migraine, and Other Disorders for Better Health*, Wiley, 1994.

Gay Hendricks, *Conscious Breathing: Breathwork for Health, Stress Release, and Personal Mastery*, Shambhala, 2012.

Wim Hof and Koen de Jong, *The Way of the Iceman: How the Wim Hof Method Creates Radiant Long-Term Health Using the Science and Secrets of Breath Control, Cold Training and Commitment*, Dragon Door Publications, 2017.

Wim Hof and Justin Rosales, *Becoming the Iceman: Pushing Past Perceived Limits*, Mill City Press, Inc., 2011.

B. K. S. Iyengar, *Light on Pranayama: The Yogic Art of Breathing*, Crossroad Publishing Company, 1985.

Swami Rama, Rudolph Ballentine, MD, and Alan Hymes, MD, *The Science of Breath—A Practical Guide*, Himalayan Institute Press, new edition, 2007.

Swami Niranjananananda Saraswati, *Prana and Pranayama*, Bihar School of Yoga/Yoga Publications Trust/Munger, 2010.

Swami Saradananda, *The Power of Breath: Yoga Breathing for Inner Balance, Health and Harmony*, Watkins Publishing, 2017.

Yogi Ramacharaka, *Science of Breath: A Complete Manual of the Oriental Breathing Philosophy of Physical, Mental, Psychic and Spiritual Development*, Watchmaker Publishing, 2011.

Performance Breathwork

Patrick McKeown, *The Oxygen Advantage: The Simple Scientifically Proven Breathing Technique That Will Revolutionise Your Health and Fitness*, Piatkus, 2015.

Vladimir Yasiliev with Scott Meredith, *Let Every Breath: Secrets of the Russian Breath Masters*, Russian Martial Art, 2006.

Other Reading

Dr. Joe Dispenza, *Breaking the Habit of Being Yourself: How to Lose Your Mind and Create a New One*, Hay House Inc., reprint edition, 2013.

Stephen Porges, *The Pocket Guide to the Polyvagal Theory: The Transformative Power of Feeling Safe*, W. W. Norton & Company, 2017.

Stanley Rosenberg, *Accessing the Healing Power of the Vagus Nerve: Self-Help Exercises for Anxiety, Depression, Trauma and Autism*, North Atlantic Books, 2017.

John E. Sarno, MD, *The Divided Mind: The Epidemic of Mindbody Disorders*, Harper Perennial, 2007.

Bessel van der Kolk, MD, *The Body Keeps the Score: Brain, Mind, and Body in the Healing of Trauma*, Penguin Books, reprint edition, 2015.

Index